RADIOLOGY CASES FOR
MEDICAL STUDENT OSCEs

RADIOLOGY CASES FOR MEDICAL STUDENT OSCEs

DEBBIE WAI,
RAKESH P PATEL,
KAREN ATKIN AND
SHAHID HUSSAIN

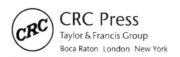

CRC Press
Taylor & Francis Group
Boca Raton London New York

CRC Press is an imprint of the
Taylor & Francis Group, an **informa** business

Radcliffe Publishing Ltd
18 Marcham Road
Abingdon
Oxon OX14 1AA
United Kingdom

www.radcliffepublishing.com
Electronic catalogue and worldwide online ordering facility.

British Library Cataloguing in Publication Data

A catalogue record for this book is available from the British Library.

ISBN-13: 978 184619 452 8

The paper used for the text pages of this book
is FSC certified. FSC (The Forest Stewardship
Council) is an international network to promote
responsible management of the world's forests.

Typeset by Phoenix Photosetting, Chatham, Kent

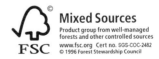

Mixed Sources
Product group from well-managed
forests and other controlled sources
www.fsc.org Cert no. SGS-COC-2482
© 1996 Forest Stewardship Council
FSC

Contents

Preface

Recent advances in imaging have meant that clinical radiology is now integral to the management of almost all patients. There is increasing awareness of radiology teaching in medical schools. The specialty now forms part of the core curriculum and radiology is now assessed in the final medical OSCE. Our book addresses this progression and includes 100 radiology cases that medical students are likely to encounter in their exams.

The book is primarily image based and includes up-to-date modalities such as CT and MRI. Particular focus has been placed on helping the medical student in the recognition and interpretation of abnormal image findings.

We hope this book will serve as an invaluable aid for candidates of the final year medical examination as well as a useful aid for junior doctors.

Debbie Wai
Rakesh P Patel
Karen Atkin
Shahid Hussain
June 2010

About the authors

Debbie Wai completed her medical degree at the University of Birmingham, United Kingdom in 2005. She then went on to work as a Foundation doctor in the West Midlands area, before taking up a place on the West Midlands Radiology Training scheme. She is currently a specialist registrar in radiology in the West Midlands. Her subspecialty interests include Chest and Musculoskeletal imaging. She is a co-author on a session for the Radiology Integrated Training Initiative. Debbie has also taught radiological anatomy to medical students from Warwick University. Other interests include website design.

Rakesh P Patel studied medicine at The Barts and The London School of Medicine and Dentistry and did an intercalated BSc in Physiology with accounting and management at King's College London. After graduating in 2003, Rakesh underwent Basic Surgical Training in London and became a Member of the Royal College of Surgeons before commencing his training in Clinical Radiology. Rakesh is currently working as a specialist registrar in the West Midlands training scheme, his areas of special interest include interventional radiology and musculoskeletal radiology. In addition to his career in radiology, Rakesh has gained formal qualifications in Information Technology and has been involved in the development and implementation of several medical IT projects on a global scale.

Karen Atkin is currently a final year registrar in radiology in the West Midlands, with subspecialty interests in Paediatric and Gynaecological imaging. She graduated from the University of Manchester in 2000, initially training in general medicine and gaining MRCP (UK) in 2003. In 2005 she commenced her radiology training in Birmingham, passing final FRCR examinations in 2008. Karen enjoys teaching and has been involved with radiology teaching of medical students from both Birmingham and Warwick universities. For the last three years she has also held Honorary Clinical Tutor status at the University of Birmingham School of Medicine, with a role of personal mentor to a group of medical students.

Shahid Hussain completed his medical degree at the University of Cambridge, United Kingdom. He is a member of the Royal College of Physicians and a Fellow of the Royal College of Radiologists. Shahid carried out his radiology training on the West Midlands training scheme, with subspecialist cardiac imaging training at the Harefield and Brompton NHS Trust. He is currently working as a Cardiothoracic

Consultant Radiologist with interest in lung cancer, interstitial lung disease, cardiac CT and MRI, at the Heart of England NHS Foundation Teaching Trust. He is the Cardiothoracic Radiology Lead for the West Midlands Training scheme. Shahid is also an author on several other books including *Radiology MCQs for the New FRCR 2A* and *Rapid Review of Radiology*.

Acknowledgements

We would like to thank our colleagues below for their contribution of images:
Dr Arvind Pallan, Dr Ben Miller, Dr Mike Pitt, Dr Philippa Skippage, Dr Nadya Polunin, Dr Gordon Jones

We would also like to thank the following hospitals for their contributions:
The Royal Orthopaedic Hospital, Birmingham
Sandwell and City Hospitals, Birmingham

Chapter 1
Introduction

Radiology continues to play an ever increasing role in the practice of medicine, in all specialties. Nearly every patient will undergo some form of imaging examination during the investigation and treatment of their complaint, and it is essential that all doctors have a basic knowledge of imaging and its techniques in order to best investigate and manage their patients.

The undergraduate medical curriculum should provide a core knowledge of radiology that will enable the newly qualified doctor to be competent and to feel confident in interpreting X-rays in the context of the clinical setting in which they are requesting them. They should also be aware of the role of more complex imaging examinations such as CT and MRI, their pros and cons, and why these examinations are likely to help them to answer a clinical question.

Methods of teaching radiology in the undergraduate curriculum will vary between medical schools, but radiological image interpretation is increasingly being assessed in OSCE examinations from year one (where radiological images can often be used to test anatomy knowledge), to year five (where interpretation of an abdominal or chest X-ray may be a station in a finals OSCE).

The cases included in this book aim to provide the student with a wide variety of radiological case examples across the specialties, with an emphasis on the interpretation of chest and abdominal plain films in the context of common clinical scenarios likely to be encountered during their first year working as a doctor (or during their final examinations)! A short discussion about the case follows, either concentrating on the disease process that has resulted in the imaging findings, or focusing on important aspects of the imaging findings, differential diagnosis or technique used. CT and MRI images are included for illustration and comparison. We also recognise that although some conditions are rarely encountered in a clinical setting, they have a relatively high incidence and prevalence in medical examinations, and some of these cases have also been included!

A systematic approach to image interpretation is essential, and should always be performed with the clinical setting in mind. Remember that the image is always easier to interpret following a thorough history and clinical examination. Image interpretation relies heavily on pattern recognition and so the more you see, the more confident you will feel in your interpretation. Perhaps the most important thing to remember is that there is always someone to ask if you are unsure. Be confident, but aware of your limitations and remember that if you have not seen anything like it before... ask for a second opinion.

We hope that you find the book educational and enjoyable.

Chapter 2
Basic physics

Clinical radiologists employ a variety of imaging modalities including plain film radiography, computed tomography (CT), ultrasound, magnetic resonance imaging (MRI), and nuclear imaging. The basic physics of each of these modalities will be described in this chapter.

PRODUCTION OF X-RAYS

An X-ray tube consists of 2 electrodes (an anode and a cathode) sealed in a vacuum. In the production of X-rays, the cathode is heated to high temperatures causing it to emit electrons. The electrons are accelerated towards the anode, due to a high potential difference between the cathode and anode. As the electrons strike the anode, a percentage of the kinetic energy is converted into X-rays.

X-ray photons are attenuated (absorbed or scattered) as they interact with matter. The amount of attenuation depends on the density of the material, atomic number of the material and photon energy. The greater the density of material and the greater the atomic number of the material, the greater the attenuation of the X-ray beam. The greater the photon energy, the lower the attenuation of the X-ray beam.

The more the X-ray beam is attenuated, the fewer the number of X-ray photons that leaves the patient and strikes the film, and the less blackening of the film that occurs. Materials that attenuate the beam significantly are referred to as radio-opaque materials, due to the white appearance of the film. Materials that do not attenuate the beam significantly are referred to as radio-lucent, due to the black appearance of the film. There are four types of radiographic densities: air, fat, water and metal. These appear as black, grey-black, grey and white, respectively.

COMPUTED TOMOGRAPHY

CT scanning was invented by the British inventor Sir Godfrey Hounsfield in the 1970s. The original CT scanners involve an X-ray tube and detector system mounted on a rotating frame or gantry, which is rotated 360 degrees around the patient. Several X-ray beams from different angles are passed simultaneously through the patient. The intensity of radiation leaving the patient is measured by the detectors. A transverse slice of the patient is imaged and cross-sectional two dimensional images are generated.

The newer spiral (helical) CT scanner uses slip ring technology which allows electric power to be transferred from a stationary power source onto a continuously rotating gantry. There is continuous rotation of the X-ray tube and simultaneous steady movement of the table with the acquisition of a volume of data, allowing faster scanning.

NUCLEAR IMAGING

Nuclear imaging utilises unstable nuclei (radionuclides). Technetium is the most commonly used radionuclide. Radionuclides decay with the emission of alpha, beta and gamma radiation. In nuclear imaging, a radionuclide is combined with a chemical compound (forming a radiopharmaceutical) to ensure selective uptake and concentration by certain tissues or organs. The radiopharmaceutical can be injected intravenously or given orally and its location is signalled by the emission of gamma rays. Gamma rays have identical properties to X-rays. The gamma rays are collected by a gamma camera, forming an image. Nuclear medicine diagnostic imaging differs from CT and MRI because it primarily evaluates function, rather than anatomy.

ULTRASOUND

Ultrasound utilises sound waves (which are not part of the electromagnetic spectrum). The ultrasound waves are emitted by a transducer, which converts electric energy into sound waves. Reflections or echoes of the ultrasound beam at the interface between two different media, e.g. tissue–air, are received by the transducer, converting the ultrasound waves back into electrical energy, producing an image. Ultrasound is suited for the investigations of soft tissues and in determining cystic from solid structures. It is also useful in situations where the biological hazards of radiation are to be avoided, e.g. pregnancy and children. Ultrasound permits 'real time' imaging and Doppler evaluation of blood vessels. Ultrasound imaging is non-ionising, a relatively low cost method of imaging, portable and may be used for interventional procedures making it a very useful imaging modality. However, ultrasound is user dependent and ultrasonic waves penetrate poorly through air and bone.

MAGNETIC RESONANCE IMAGING

With magnetic resonance imaging, a strong magnetic field is created around the patient. The human body contains many water molecules, each of which contains two hydrogen nuclei (protons). When the patient lies in the MRI scanner, the protons align themselves in the external magnetic field. A pulsed radiofrequency beam is sent to the patient, disturbing and re-orientating the protons relative to the magnetic field. When the radiofrequency beam is turned off, the nuclei return to their original alignment, regenerating radio waves, which are detected by the scanner, producing an image. MRI provides much greater soft tissue contrast than CT and is widely used in imaging of the neurological, cardiovascular and musculoskeletal systems.

THE BIOLOGICAL EFFECT OF RADIATION

An atom is ionised when one of its electrons has been completely removed. X-rays and gamma-rays cause ionisation of atoms of living cells causing biological damage.

Damage to DNA, RNA and enzymes leads ultimately leads to cell death, inhibition of cell division or transformation to a malignant state. The period of time between radiation exposure and the detection of cancer can be many years. X-rays and gamma rays are part of the electromagnetic spectrum and are ionising radiations. MRI and ultrasound do not produce ionising radiation.

The chest X-ray is one of the lowest radiation exposure medical examinations performed. High dose procedures include CT scan of the abdomen and barium enemas, *see* Table 2.1.

Table 2.1 Comparison of radiation doses of diagnostic procedures.

Diagnostic procedure	Typical effective dose (mSv)	Number of equivalent chest X-rays (PA film)
Chest X-ray (PA film)	0.02	1
Skull X-ray	0.1	5
Lumbar spine	1.5	75
Upper GI exam	6	300
Barium enema	8	400
CT head	2	100
CT abdomen	8	400

It is important to consider the best imaging modality in each specific clinical situation. In certain situations, non-ionising radiation imaging methods such ultrasound and/or MRI may be considered as the first line. Examples of which are:

- **suspected gall bladder disease** – ultrasound is the investigation of choice to show or to exclude gallstones and acute cholecystitis. It is the initial investigation of biliary pain but cannot reliably exclude common duct stones. CT has a limited role in cholelithiasis but is useful in assessment of the gallbladder wall and gall-bladder masses
- **suspected pelvic mass** – a combination of transabdominal and transvaginal ultra-sound is often required. MRI is the best second line investigation
- **renal failure** – ultrasound is indicated as the first investigation to measure kidney size and parenchymal thickness and to check for pelvicalyceal dilatation indicating possible obstruction.

FURTHER READING

- The Royal College of Radiologists. *Making the best use of clinical radiology services (MBUR).* 6th ed. London: Royal College of Radiologists; 2007.

Chapter 3
Approaching a film

It is essential as a junior doctor to be able to interpret chest and abdominal radiographs since these are often still the first line imaging investigation in the acute setting. The junior doctor is also frequently the first one to look at these films! A good knowledge of chest/abdominal radiological anatomy coupled with a systematic approach to the film will ensure that pathology is identified and a correct diagnosis can be reached.

APPROACHING A CHEST RADIOGRAPH

When examining a chest radiograph, a systematic approach should be employed and the following factors should be first considered.

General points
- Name, age, sex of the patient (look for breast shadows).
- Left and right markers (beware of dextrocardia).
- Is the film a posteroanterior (PA), anteroposterior (AP) film or lateral view? (With a PA film, the scapulae are thrown off the chest. Another subtle clue is that the upper thoracic spinous processes are sharper on a PA film and the vertebral end-plates are sharper on an AP film.)
- Is there a marker to indicate whether the film was taken in inspiration or expiration? (A chest X-ray may be taken in expiration if performed for a suspected pneumothorax.)
- Are there any markings to indicate whether the film was taken erect, semi-supine or supine? (The chest X-ray may be taken erect if performed for suspected air beneath the diaphragm. The chest X-ray may be taken supine if the patient is very unwell.)
- Is the patient sitting upright or leaning over to one side (may be too unwell to sit up).
- Are there ECG wires, tubing, and/or an oxygen mask to suggest the patient is unwell?
- Are there any previous films or is this a single film?

Quality of the film
- Rotation – the distance between the medial aspects of each clavicle and spinous processes should be equidistant.

- Penetration – at least one vertebra should be visible behind the heart.
- Inspiration – the anterior aspects of at least six ribs should be visible above the left dome of the diaphragm for an adequate inspiration.

BASIC ANATOMY OF THE CHEST

It is important to be familiar with the basic anatomy of the chest in order to be able to recognise normal structures and localise disease.

- There are three lobes in the right lung (upper, middle and lower) and two lobes in the left lung (upper and lower).
- The oblique fissure separates the right upper lobe and right middle lobe from the right lower lobe.
- Similarly, the left upper lobe is separated from the left lower lobe by the oblique fissure.
- The right upper lobe is separated from the right middle lobe by the horizontal fissure which is approximately at the level of the right hilum. The corresponding lobe in the left lung is called the lingula.

The lobes of each lung are illustrated in Figures 3.1, 3.2 and 3.3.

- The hilar points are the angles formed by the superior pulmonary veins as they cross the right and left lower lobe pulmonary arteries.
- The left hilum should be higher than the right. They may occasionally be at the same level in some individuals.
- The right hemidiaphragm is usually 2–3 cm higher than the left.

On the frontal chest radiograph, the cardiac silhouette can be identified as a series of 'bumps', *see* Figure 3.4.

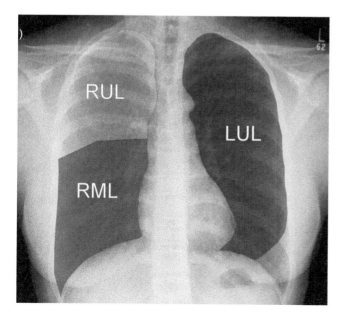

Figure 3.1 Lobar anatomy. Right middle and upper lobes, left upper lobe.

7

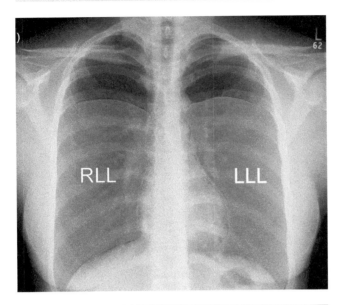

Figure 3.2 Lobar anatomy. Right and left lower lobes.

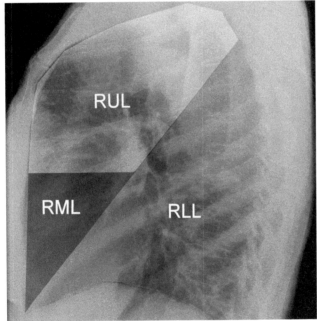

Figure 3.3 Lobar anatomy on a lateral chest radiograph.

SYSTEMIC REVIEW OF A CHEST X-RAY

Once all the general factors outlined earlier have been considered, assess the following:

- heart size (cardiothoracic ratio should be <50%)
- mediastinal contour
- lungs (compare upper, mid and lower zones)
- hila (assess position, density, size)

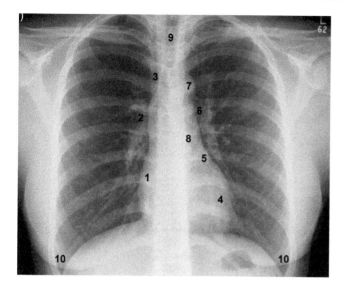

Figure 3.4 Cardiac silhouette on a chest radiograph. 1 Right atrium; 2 Right hilum; 3 SVC; 4 Left ventricle; 5 Left atrial appendage; 6 Left hilum; 7 Aortic arch; 8 Descending aorta; 9 Trachea; 10 Costophrenic angle.

- diaphragm
- costophrenic angles
- bones (look at each rib, clavicles, scapulae, humeral heads) and soft tissues.

The following are useful review areas to remember if the chest X-ray appears normal:

- lung apices
- beneath the diaphragm
- behind the heart and descending aorta
- along the pleura
- hila again!

APPROACHING AN ABDOMINAL RADIOGRAPH

When examining an abdominal radiograph, a systematic approach should be employed and the following factors should be first considered.

General points
- Name, sex and age of the patient (certain pathologies are more likely at different ages).
- Is the film a supine, erect or decubitus view?
- Left and right markers (beware of situs inversus).
- Are there any previous films or is this a single film?

Radiographic densities
There are five radiographic densities. Familiarity with these different densities will help in the interpretation of any radiograph:

1 air – gas appears black
2 fat – fat appears dark grey
3 water – soft tissue is largely made up of water and appears light grey

4   bone – calcium appears as white
5   metal – metal appears as intense white.

Air
- Stomach – in the supine position, gas is usually seen in the antrum and body of the stomach.
- Small bowel – is usually located centrally in the abdomen. Valvulae conniventes may be visible which are lines traversing across the whole diameter. Valvulae conniventes are more frequent in the proximal small bowel and decrease in frequency along its length. The calibre of the small bowel should not exceed 3 cm.
- Large bowel – is usually located peripherally in the abdomen. Haustra which are folds which do not transverse the whole diameter may be seen. The caecum may be mottled in appearance due to faeces and gas. The calibre of the large bowel should not exceed 5.5 cm. The thickness of the bowel wall in a normally distended section of bowel should not measure greater than 3 mm.
- It is worth understanding that in the supine position with the patient lying on his/her back, gas in the bowel will rise to the anterior aspect of the patient. Fluid will sink to the most dependent, posterior aspect of the patient.

Fat
- Intra-abdominal fat outlines the liver, spleen, kidneys, psoas muscle and bladder.
- Obliteration of fat planes may indicate inflammatory change, haemorrhage or tumour in that area. For example, obliteration of the right psoas margin may indicate inflammation of the fat surrounding the appendix.

Soft tissues
- Kidneys – the left kidney usually lies slightly higher than the right.
- Liver – appears as a large soft tissue density in the right upper quadrant.
- Spleen – appears as a soft tissue mass in the left upper quadrant. It is often not visible on an abdominal X-ray.
- Urinary bladder – this may be seen as a soft tissue density in the pelvis.

Causes of abdominal calcifications
- 80% to 90% of renal stones may be calcified and visible on plain film.
- Only 15% to 20% of gallstones are radio-opaque on plain film.
- Phleboliths (calcification within a vein).
- Calcified mesenteric lymph nodes.
- Appendicolith (calcified deposit in the appendix).
- Vascular calcification (an abdominal aortic aneurysm may be visible due to calcification of the wall).
- Calcification in chronic pancreatitis.

Metal
Metallic objects may be present on an abdominal radiograph, and should be examined for closely. For example:

- surgical staples (usually centrally in the midline)

- metallic stents
- sterilisation clips in the pelvis.

On the supine abdominal radiograph, Figure 3.5, the following structures can be identified:

1 liver
2 kidneys
3 psoas muscle
4 ascending colon
5 descending colon
6 phlebolith
7 properitoneal fat
8 spleen

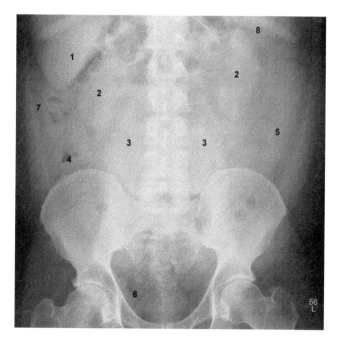

Figure 3.5 Structures identified on an abdominal radiograph.

SYSTEMIC REVIEW OF AN ABDOMINAL X-RAY

- Is there any abnormal gas?
- Bowel (position, diameter).
- Bowel wall thickness.
- Assess for pneumoperitoneum (if indicated in clinical history).
- Soft tissues (liver, renal, spleen). Is there organomegaly or displacement?
- Are the psoas muscles clearly outlined?
- Is there any abnormal calcification? (Abdominal aorta, splenic artery calcification, renal calculi, appendicolith.)
- Bones (pelvis, spine, sacroiliac joints, proximal femora, ribs). Are there any degenerative changes, evidence of malignancy?
- Lung bases (do not miss a cancer at the lung base)!

Case 1

A 70-year-old man complains of fever, cough, dyspnoea and left sided chest pain. On examination, there are crepitations at the left base. A chest X-ray is obtained.

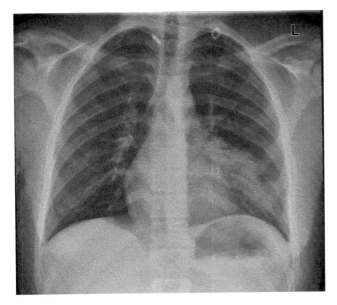

Figure 1.1

Image findings: the chest X-ray shows that the left heart border is indistinct. There is air space opacification in the left mid to lower zones. An air-filled bronchus can be seen within this area of shadowing. This patient has a consolidation in the lingula. Notice how the left hemidiaphragm is clearly seen, indicating that the pneumonia is not affecting the left lower lobe. The right lung is clear. The symptoms point to infection as the cause of consolidation.

Diagnosis: lingula consolidation.

ANATOMY

There are two lobes in the left lung, the upper lobe and the lower lobe. These are separated by the oblique fissure. The homologue of the right middle lobe is called the lingula. The upper lobe has four segments: apicoposterior, anterior, superior lingula and inferior lingula. The left lower lobe has four segments and consists of: apical, anterior basal, posterior basal and lateral basal segments. The lingula lies in anatomic contact with the left heart border and disease here will obliterate this border. The silhouette sign can be used to explain this phenomenon.

THE SILHOUETTE SIGN

Anatomic structures are recognised on the chest X-ray because of their different densities. On a normal chest X-ray the well-defined borders of the heart and diaphragm are visualised because the adjacent lung provides an interface. Two similar densities in contact with each other will obliterate the existing interface. Pneumonia (water density) abutting the heart (water density) will obliterate that border. The loss of the normal silhouette of a border of the heart, aorta or diaphragm, is known as the silhouette sign, *see* Figure 1.2.

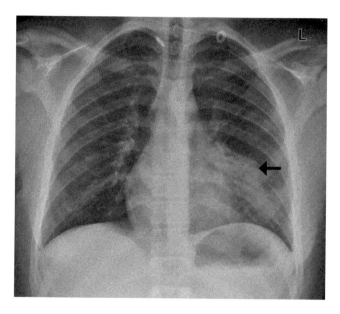

Figure 1.2 Chest radiograph showing poor definition of the left heart border due to consolidation in the region of the lingula (arrow).

AIR BRONCHOGRAM

Normal bronchi are not visible on a chest X-ray because:

- they contain air and are surrounded by air in the alveoli
- they have very thin walls.

The visualisation of air in the bronchi is known as an air bronchogram. This can occur, as in this case, because the air filled bronchus is surrounded by water density (pneumonia).

Case 2

A 70-year-old man, who is a retired ship builder, is admitted for elective hernia repair. A CXR is performed as part of pre-operative assessment due to mild shortness of breath on exertion.

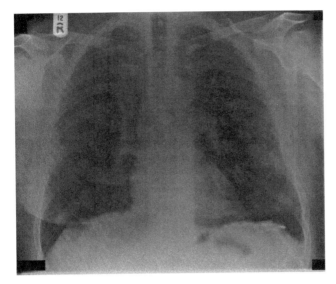

Figure 2.1

Image findings: the chest radiograph shows heavy calcification over both hemidiaphragms. There are also sharply defined 'holly leaf' configuration calcific densities overlying the lungs bilaterally. Pleural thickening is seen at the left lateral chest wall. All of these areas represent pleural plaques, many of them calcified. These are due to previous asbestos exposure.

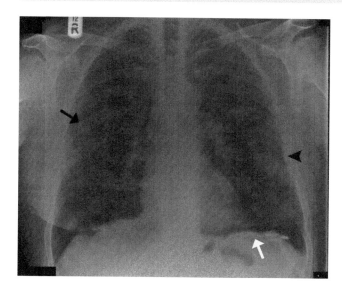

Figure 2.2 Chest radiograph showing a 'holly leaf' configuration of a pleural plaque on the anterior pleural surface (black arrow), pleural thickening (arrowhead) and calcification over the diaphragm (white arrow).

Diagnosis: calcified pleural plaques.

Asbestos related lung disease remains an important health issue, despite the reduction in asbestos use in the United Kingdom, due to the long latency (often >15yrs) between exposure to the substance and development of disease. There are several types of asbestos – crocidolite (blue/black) asbestos is associated with the most severe disease. A detailed occupational history is essential. The chest diseases associated with asbestos exposure are:

- benign pleural plaque disease (as seen in this case)
- asbestosis – this is lung fibrosis secondary to asbestos exposure. The fibrosis is usually worse in the lower zones of the lungs
- malignant mesothelioma – asbestos exposure increases the risk × 30. In asbestos workers, 10% will develop this fatal malignancy
- lung cancer – asbestos increases the risk × 5.

The causes of pleural calcification include:

- calcified pleural plaques
- calcification post resolution of a tuberculosis empyema
- calcification post resolution of a haemothorax
- post pleurodesis.

Case 3

A 62-year-old lady presents with worsening shortness of breath over the past two weeks, and a productive cough, sometimes coughing up blood.

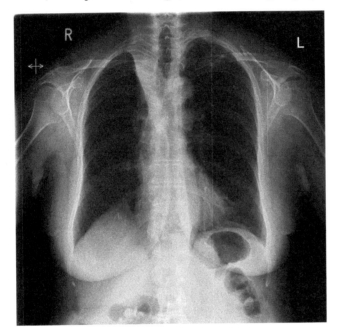

Figure 3.1

Image findings: the chest radiograph shows a very well demarcated 'wedge shaped', dense opacity in the right upper zone adjacent to the right superior mediastinum. There is a reduction in right lung volume, the trachea is pulled slightly to the right, and the right hemidiaphragm is pulled upward ('tented'). This appearance is of right upper lobe collapse.

Diagnosis: right upper lobe collapse.

Lobar collapse is an important feature to identify on the chest radiograph. It occurs due to the occlusion of a central bronchus, and the most common cause of this, in the middle-aged to elderly population, is an occluding bronchogenic carcinoma. For this reason further investigation with either CT or bronchoscopy is essential in this group of patients to exclude a neoplasm, *see* Figure 3.2.

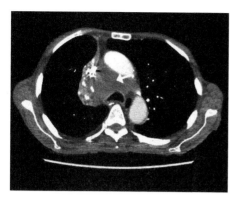

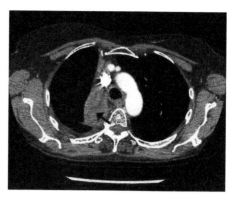

Figure 3.2 Axial CT image demonstrating a soft tissue mediastinal mass (white arrow) causing complete collapse of the right upper lobe.

Figure 3.3 Axial CT image showing the right upper lobe collapsing medially (arrow).

In younger adults or children, mucus plugging secondary to asthma is the commonest cause, whilst in the younger child foreign body inhalation can lead to lobar collapse (most often lower lobe).

Right upper lobe collapse has specific features as demonstrated by this case. On the frontal chest radiograph, the right upper lobe occupies the right upper zone, with its inferior aspect demarcated by the right horizontal fissure. When the right upper lobe collapses, the right horizontal fissure moves 'like a clock hand' on the chest X-ray, from a 9 o'clock to 11 o'clock position, resulting in a 'wedge' of collapsed right upper lobe abutting the superior mediastinum.

Case 4

A 78-year-old man presents to accident and emergency with central chest pain radiating to his left arm, and shortness of breath. He is coughing up pink frothy sputum. On examination the man is clammy and sweating with a raised respiratory rate of 25 breaths per minute. Crepitations can be heard in the mid and lower zones of both lungs, and there is dullness to percussion at both lung bases.

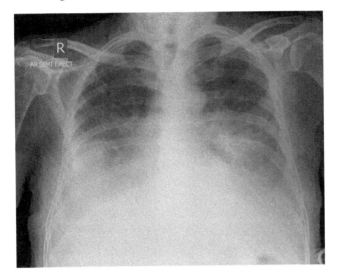

Figure 4.1

Image findings: the chest radiograph shows shadowing in the regions surrounding both hila. This peri-hilar shadowing is known as a 'bat's-wing' distribution, and is characteristic for pulmonary oedema (although not all that commonly seen). There is denser shadowing in the lower zones bilaterally, with loss of definition of the hemidiaphragms, in keeping with bilateral pleural effusions. This is a case of pulmonary oedema due to acute myocardial infarction.

Diagnosis: heart failure.

Pulmonary oedema is a fairly common finding in myocardial infarction. It occurs due to left ventricular failure and resulting increased pulmonary venous and capillary hydrostatic pressure. As the pressure increases there is enlargement of the pulmonary veins and 'diversion' of pulmonary blood flow from the lower lobes to the upper lobes. This 'upper lobe blood diversion' can be the first sign on the CXR. The upper lobe blood vessels are seen to be of larger diameter than the lower lobe (reversal of the normal pattern). As pressure increases fluid leaks from the capillaries into the pulmonary interstitium (interstitial oedema) where it is seen as thickened interstitial markings on the CXR (Kerley lines). The most commonly identified of these are Kerley B (septal) lines, seen as horizontal white lines in the costophrenic recesses.

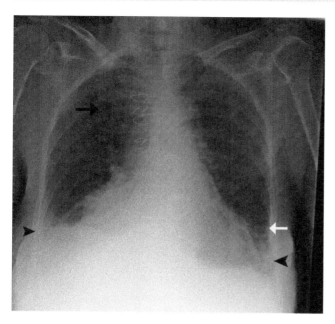

Figure 4.2 Chest radiograph showing central sternotomy wires in a patient who has had a previous coronary artery bypass graft surgery for triple vessel disease. There is cardiomegaly and there are features of heart failure with an increase in size of the upper zone pulmonary vascularity due to pulmonary congestion (black arrow), blunting of the costophrenic angles due to bilateral small pleural effusions (arrowheads) and Kerley B lines due to interstitial oedema (white arrow).

Eventually the interstitium becomes full of fluid, which then spills over into the air spaces (alveoli), resulting in the bilateral airspace shadowing seen in this case.

There are several cardiac causes of heart failure which include ischaemia, infarction, cardiomyopathy, myocarditis, valvular heart disease and infiltrative disease, e.g. sarcoid, amyloid. Heart failure is usually clinically classified using the New York Heart Association Classification which helps to guide treatment.

- Class I – no limitation of physical activity.
- Class II – slight limitation and symptoms on ordinary activity. No symptoms at rest.
- Class III – marked limitation of activity with symptoms occurring at less than ordinary activity.
- Class IV – severe limitation. Symptoms at rest.

Echocardiography and cardiac MRI are useful in assessing cardiac function and determining the left ventricular ejection fraction. Treatment is primarily pharmacological with diuretics, vasodilators and ACE inhibitors. In more advanced disease there is a role for ventricular resynchronisation devices, implantable defibrillators and cardiac transplant.

It should be remembered that left ventricular failure is only one cause of pulmonary oedema. Other causes include fluid overload, neurogenic causes (stroke, head injury), drugs/poisons, and adult respiratory distress syndrome (ARDS).

Case 5

A 27-year-old female with a long history of respiratory problems since childhood presented to her general practitioner (GP) with worsening shortness of breath and cough productive of green sputum.

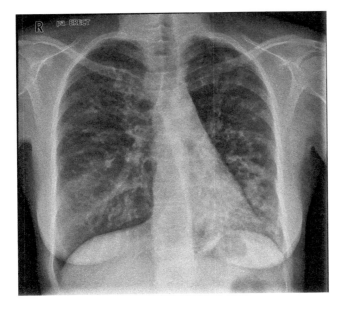

Figure 5.1

Image findings: the chest radiograph shows extensive reticular (lines) and ring shadowing throughout both lungs. The parallel reticular markings or 'tram-tracks' represent the thickened walls of dilated bronchi, whilst the ring shadows represent the thick walled, dilated bronchi seen 'en face'. The lung volumes are normal to hyper-expanded. These features are of bronchiectasis, in this case due to cystic fibrosis. In the left lower zone there is additional patchy air space shadowing which is likely due to acute infection which has led to the deterioration in the clinical condition.

Diagnosis: cystic fibrosis.

Bronchiectasis is defined as irreversible dilatation of the bronchi which are thickened and subsequently act as foci for recurrent infections. There are multiple causes of bronchiectasis which include:
- congenital – cystic fibrosis, Kartagener's syndrome
- post infection – TB, measles, whooping cough, Swyer–James syndrome, allergic bronchopulmonary aspergillosis
- distal to an obstruction – tumour, foreign body
- aspiration

- lung fibrosis (the fibrosis pulls the bronchi open resulting in a 'traction bronchiectasis').

The findings in bronchiectasis are very well demonstrated by CT, where the dilated thick walled bronchi are more clearly visualised, *see* Figure 5.2.

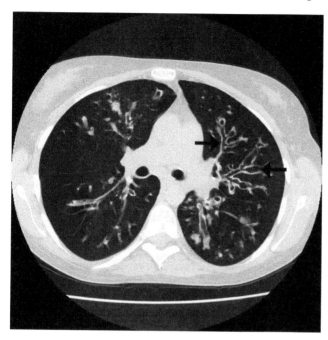

Figure 5.2 Axial CT image showing the thick walled dilated bronchi in the mid zones bilaterally (arrows) in a patient with bronchiectasis.

Cystic fibrosis is an autosomal recessive inherited condition that results in abnormal thick mucus secretions. The defective gene is sited on chromosome seven, and the gene is carried by approximately 1 in 20 Caucasians. Diagnosis is confirmed by measuring the sodium concentration in sweat (>70 mmol/l in children). The abnormal mucus blocks exocrine ducts and causes damage to multiple organs including the lungs, gastrointestinal tract (GIT) and pancreas. The disease often manifests soon after birth with failure to pass meconium (meconium ileus). In children it presents with:

- lungs – recurrent chest infections (thick mucus causes recurrent blockage of the small airways which explains the cycles of recurrent infections from birth), bronchiectasis, recurrent pneumothoraces
- gastrointestinal – distal intestinal obstruction
- pancreas – pancreatic failure, recurrent pancreatitis, diabetes mellitus (DM)
- liver – fatty liver, portal hypertension
- gallbladder – gallstones.

Pulmonary complications are the commonest cause of morbidity and death.

Case 6

A 63-year-old lady presented to her general practitioner with longstanding epigastric discomfort and retrosternal 'burning', particularly after eating.

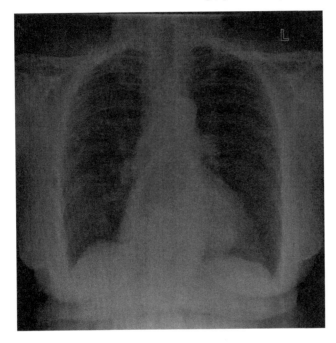

Figure 6.1

Image findings: the chest radiograph shows a large mass projected over the heart in the midline, containing an air bubble and an air/fluid level. Note is made that the gastric bubble is **not** seen in its normal position below the left hemidiaphragm. The lungs are clear. This appearance is that of a large hiatus hernia, with the majority of the stomach sited within the thorax. Previous X-rays are often very useful for comparison when in doubt about the diagnosis, as these have often been present for a long time.

Diagnosis: hiatus hernia.

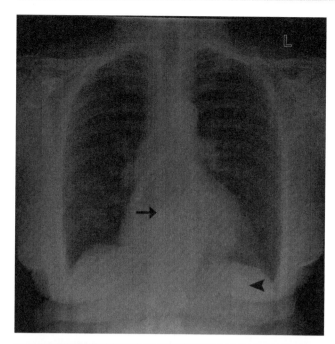

Figure 6.2 Chest radiograph demonstrating a mass behind the heart, with an air fluid level (arrow) due to a hiatus hernia. Note that a gastric bubble is not seen in its normal position (arrowhead).

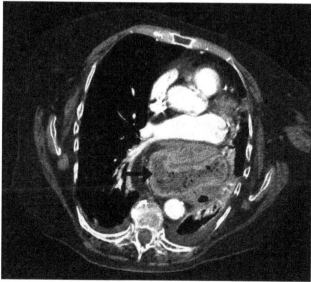

Figure 6.3 Axial CT image showing a large hiatus hernia with most of the stomach lying within the chest cavity (arrow).

A hiatus hernia is a very common abnormality but it can cause confusion if not correctly identified on the chest radiograph. They are categorised into two groups, sliding and rolling.

In a sliding hernia the gastro-oesophageal junction slides up through the oesophageal hiatus to lie above the diaphragm.

In a rolling (or para-oesophageal) hernia, part of the stomach (usually the fundus) passes through the oesophageal hiatus alongside the oesophagus, leaving the gastro-oesophageal junction below the diaphragm.

Hiatus herniae are mostly asymptomatic, however, they are commonly associated with gastro-oesophageal reflux which can cause symptoms such as those described in this case.

It is important not to confuse a hiatus hernia with another cause of a thick walled cavity with an air fluid level behind the heart. Other important pathologies that can produce a similar radiological appearance would be:

- infection – abscess, septic embolus, infected bulla
- cavitating tumour/metastasis (squamous cell carcinomas are more likely to cavitate)
- infarction/haematoma.

Clinical history and examination is therefore very important to differentiate these from a benign cause. The radiological clue that the abnormality represents a hiatus hernia is the absence of the gastric bubble below the left hemidiaphragm since the gastric fundus is within the chest cavity!

Case 7

An 80-year-old lady presents to accident and emergency. She had been found on the floor at home by her daughter and it was presumed she had fallen. The lady suffers from dementia and is unable to give a coherent history. A few basal crepitations are heard on examination of the chest, and a CXR is therefore requested.

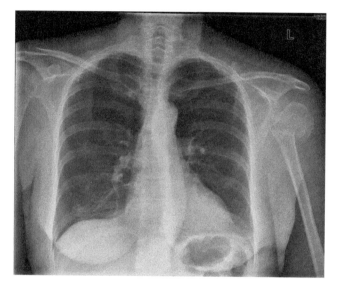

Figure 7.1

Image findings: the radiograph shows a fracture of the neck of the left humerus. The humeral head itself is subluxed, but not completely dislocated. Otherwise the chest X-ray is normal in appearance.

Diagnosis: humeral fracture.

It is important to have a system for reviewing the CXR to ensure that all areas are examined, including *all* of the bony structures and soft tissues. It is particularly important when the patient is unable to communicate areas of pain or discomfort and is unable to give a history, as in this case. It is common in an exam situation to be shown a radiograph with an abnormality at the edge of the film – when reporting any radiological image one must analyse everything on the film.

Ensure that part of your system for reviewing chest radiographs includes reviews of:

- bones, looking for: fractures, bone tumours
- soft tissues, in particular: breast shadows, axillae.

It is also useful to have a few specific review areas which are worth specifically remembering to check on every chest radiograph to ensure that you have looked at everything. These are particularly useful if you think that the chest radiograph is normal. Review areas could include:

- lung apices – looking for a small pancoast tumour
- behind the heart – a lung cancer could be missed due to the overlying heart shadow
- below the diaphragms – to exclude free gas from a perforated viscus
- along the pleural edge – for pleural thickening.

Case 8

An 11-year-old boy is an unrestrained rear seat passenger in a car involved in a head on collision with a van. In the emergency department the boy complains of chest pain. An initial chest radiograph is performed.

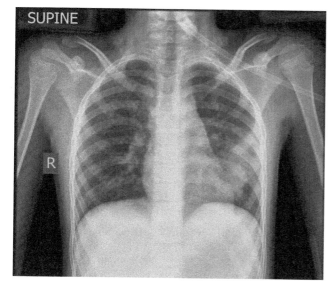

Figure 8.1

Image findings: there are bilateral fractures of the lateral aspects of the clavicles. There is also a linear fracture through the first rib on the left. No pneumothorax is seen. There is some airspace opacity seen adjacent to the left heart border slightly obscuring it – suggesting that there is pathology in the lingua. In the clinical context this would be consistent with lung haemorrhage/contusion.

Diagnosis: bilateral clavicle fractures, first rib fracture and lung contusion.

It is essential not to miss fractures of the first ribs since they are often associated with a significant impact and there is therefore likely to be significant intrathoracic trauma. These can be associated with:

- tracheal rupture
- injury to the lung characterised by lung contusion or haemorrhage
- vascular injury with laceration to the aorta – this is associated with a rapid deceleration injury, e.g. unrestrained in RTA, a fall from a height or crushing chest injury. The most common site to get a laceration is at the level of the aortic isthmus which is at the distal point of the aortic arch. This is because the brachiocephalic arteries and the ligamentum arteriosum keep the aorta in place in this region. Up to 30% of patients with an aortic injury will present with a normal CXR, so always

consider the mechanism of injury. Urgent chest CT is the next investigation of choice

- pneumothorax/haemopneumothorax
- tear to the oesophagus.

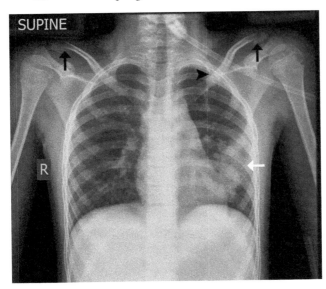

Figure 8.2 Chest radiograph revealing bilateral clavicular fractures (black arrows), fracture of the left first rib (arrowhead) and lung contusions (white arrow).

Case 9

A 62-year-old male is referred to the respiratory clinic by his general practitioner due to increasing breathlessness, weight loss and this abnormal CXR. As a young man he spent 10 years in the ship building trade in Liverpool.

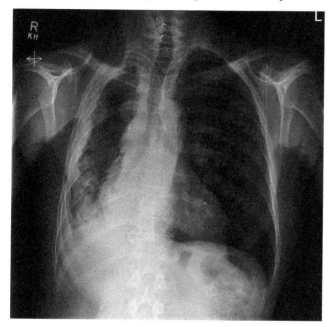

Figure 9.1

Image findings: the chest radiograph shows extensive lobulated pleural thickening encasing the right hemithorax, including over the mediastinal pleura. There is associated volume loss in the right lung and mediastinal shift towards the right. The left lung is clear, with mild compensatory hyperinflation. These findings are typical for malignant mesothelioma.

Diagnosis: malignant mesothelioma.

Malignant mesothelioma is a rare but important neoplasm which is associated with prior asbestos exposure. Unlike the benign spectrum of disease associated with asbestos (*see* Case 2), the risk of developing malignant mesothelioma does not appear to be dose related and can occur after only minimal exposure. Between 5–10% of asbestos workers will develop mesothelioma. There is often a long time lag of 30 to 40 years between the exposure and development of disease. Malignant mesothelioma carries a very poor prognosis with median survival time of approximately 6 to 12 months from diagnosis.

A haemorrhagic pleural effusion is present in the majority of patients with mesothelioma, and can be so large as to obscure much or all of the pleural thickening.

The tumour usually spreads locally to the hilar/mediastinal lymph nodes, lung and can extend through the chest wall. A good occupational history is essential. Diagnosis is usually made by surgical pleural biopsy. Metastatic adenocarcinoma is the commonest differential diagnosis and surgical biopsy is therefore required to determine the pathology – chemotherapy can be offered in these patients.

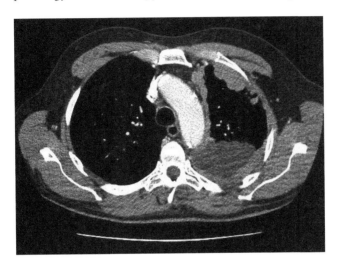

Figure 9.2 Axial CT image showing irregular lobulated pleural thickening in the left hemithorax and a large pleural effusion.

Case 10

A 55-year-old male presents to his general practitioner with a history of cough productive of sputum, on and off for the past few months. He is a long term smoker, with a family history of 'cancer' and is very anxious that he may have lung cancer. There is nothing specific to find on examination, but given the history of prolonged cough a CXR is requested.

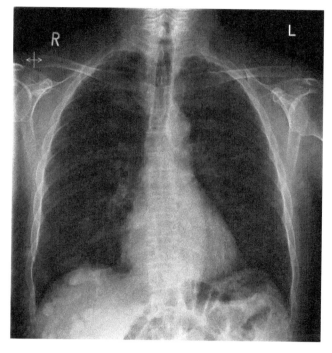

Figure 10.1

Image findings: the chest radiograph shows multiple well defined rounded opacities projected all over the thorax, with the majority of lesions seen in the right lower zone. These are projected over both the lungs and the soft tissues of the chest wall. These are typical of neurofibromata on the skin surface, in neurofibromatosis type 1.

Diagnosis: neurofibromatosis.

Neurofibromatosis type 1 (von Recklinghausen disease) is an autosomal dominantly inherited disorder with the gene located on chromosome 17. It is one of the most common inherited disorders. Clinically it is characterised by café au lait spots, neurofibromas, optic nerve gliomas, axillary freckling, Lisch nodules (iris pigmentation), and skeletal lesions (pseudoarthrosis, rib abnormalities).

Neurofibromatosis type 2 is an autosomal dominant disease located on chromosome 22. Its features include bilateral acoustic neuromas, schwannomas of other cranial nerves and multiple meningiomas.

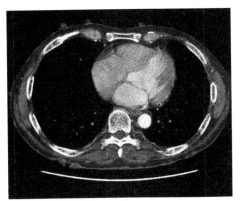 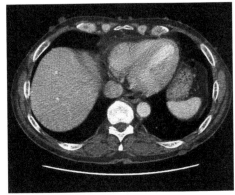

Figures 10.2 and 10.3 Axial CT images through the thorax demonstrating the cutaneous nodules (neurofibromata). The CT also confirms that there is no parenchymal lung mass.

Case 11

A 67-year-old woman presents to clinic following a single episode of haemoptysis. There is no history of cough, fever or phlegm. In her past medical history she had previously had a myocardial infarction three years ago and continued to take regular aspirin and statins. She had also had a resection of a colonic carcinoma 12 months previously. A chest X-ray is requested.

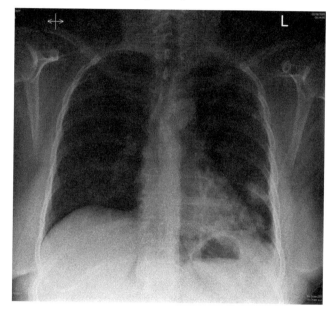

Figure 11.1

Image findings: the chest radiograph shows multiple rounded opacities of variable sizes within the left lung. These are well defined and although there are multiple causes of lung nodules, with the given clinical history, these are likely to be pulmonary metastases. Pulmonary metastases are usually smooth or lobulated lesions that are found in greater numbers in the peripheral portions of the lower lobes because of the greater pulmonary blood flow to these regions.

Diagnosis: lung metastases.

Pulmonary metastases commonly arise from tumours such as breast, colorectal, prostate, osteosarcoma, bronchial, head-and–neck, and renal. A chest X-ray is usually performed as the first investigation to detect pulmonary metastases in patients with known malignancy, however, CT has higher resolution, revealing smaller nodules, and is now recommended in the routine staging of multiple malignancies.

There are several other causes for multiple well-defined rounded lung nodules:

- neoplasia – malignant (metastases)
- infection – tuberculosis, abscesses, septic emboli
- immunological – wegener's granulomatosis, rheumatoid nodules
- vascular – arteriovenous malformations.

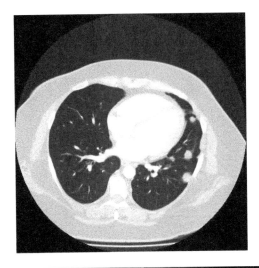

Figure 11.2 Axial CT image confirming the chest radiograph findings of multiple soft tissue nodules in the left lower lobe.

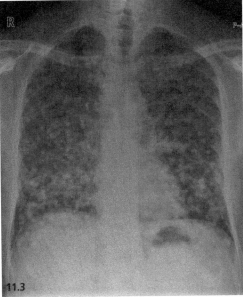

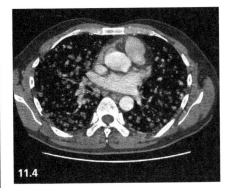

Figures 11.3 and 11.4 Chest X-ray and CT showing extensive bilateral pulmonary metastases in a patient with a thyroid tumour.

Case 12

An 80-year-old lady presents to accident and emergency complaining of dull central chest pain radiating to her left arm and neck. She has a previous history of two myocardial infarctions in the past 10 years. Her pain settles quickly with nitrates and oxygen.

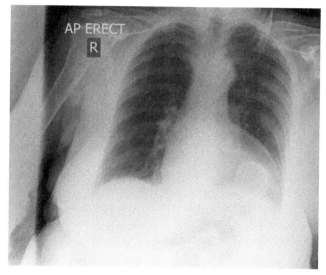

Figure 12.1

Image findings: the chest radiograph shows a well defined peripherally calcified, rounded lesion projected over the heart. It is above the left hemidiaphragm. Possibilities include a cardiac lesion or a calcified lung lesion. A CT chest was requested to help to determine the nature of the lesion.

Diagnosis: calcified left ventricular aneurysm.

There are several possible causes of a peripherally calcified chest lesion on a chest radiograph which would include:

- chronic abscess
- granuloma, e.g. TB
- pulmonary sequestration
- pulmonary hydatid
- lung infarct/haematoma
- aneurysm.

CT can be useful to better characterise the lesion and look for other abnormalities in the lung. Calcification is usually a reassuring sign in lung lesions since it suggests benignity of the lesion.

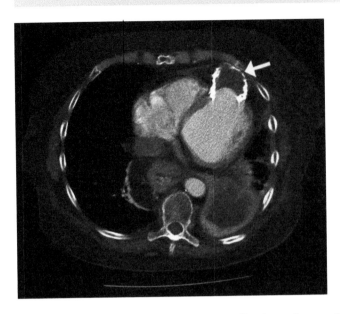

Figure 12.2 Axial CT image demonstrating the calcified left ventricular wall aneurysm with thrombus in the aneurysm (arrow).

Left ventricular aneurysms are a complication of an apical myocardial infarction. They are a reasonably rare complication which can develop four weeks or more after a myocardial infarct. The presence of heavy calcification within the wall implies that it has been present for a number of years. They can be asymptomatic (as in this case) and detected on admission for another event, however, they can also be complicated by development of thrombus within the aneurysm which can lead to systemic embolisation. They very rarely rupture. Treatment is usually by surgical resection by cardiac surgeons and this is associated with an improvement in left ventricular function.

Case 13

A 24-year-old man is a pedestrian who is knocked over by a car as he is crossing the road. When he arrives in hospital he is alert and orientated with a Glasgow Coma Scale (GCS) of 15/15. There is no amnesia and he does not black out after the event. He is however complaining of neck pain. There is no neurological deficit on examination. A cervical spine X-ray is obtained.

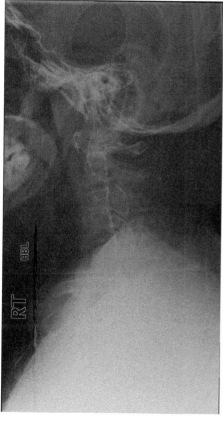

Figure 13.1

Image findings: the lateral radiograph of the cervical spine shows thickening of the soft tissues anterior to the C1 vertebral body. The maximal width of the prevertebral soft tissue should be less than one third of the width of the vertebra from C1–4 (~7 mm) and less than the width of the vertebra from C5–7 (~20–22 mm). There is significant widening of the atlantoaxial space – the distance between the anterior aspect of the odontoid peg and the posterior surface of C1 should be <3 mm (5 mm in children). In this case the distance is 8 mm. There is fracture of C1 (*see* Figure 13.2).

Diagnosis: C1 fracture.

A CT scan performed on this patient confirmed the fracture of the C1 vertebra. The widening of the peg-C1 distance suggests that there has also been rupture of the transverse ligament.

It is important when assessing trauma patients to clear the cervical spine of any injury before removing the stabilisation collar which will have been put on the patient by the paramedics. This requires both radiological and clinical assessment. Radiological assessment is usually with plain films – with an AP, lateral and odontoid peg view or by CT. On the lateral plain radiograph it is essential to ensure that the whole of the cervical spine can be seen down to the C7/T1 level. If this is not seen then manoeuvres such as pulling the shoulders down or using a swimmers view (arms elevated) can help. If sufficient coverage is still not achieved then CT is required. Systematic assessment of the films should be made for:

- prevertebral soft tissue thickness on the lateral film – as described above
- four lines of vertebral alignment – should form smooth curves on the lateral film, *see* Figure 13.4a:
  1 along the anterior margin of the vertebral bodies
  2 along the posterior margin of the vertebral bodies
  3 along the bases of the spinous processes
  4 along the tips of the spinous processes.
- spinous processes should be equidistant and in a line on the AP view, *see* Figure 13.4b.
- vertebral bodies/intervertebral disc heights should be equal
- odontoid peg position should be central with alignment of the lateral edges of C1 and C2, *see* Figure 13.4c.

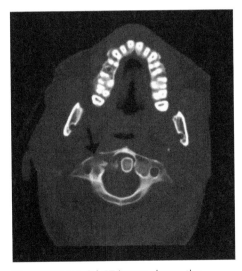

Figure 13.2 Axial CT image shows the comminuted fracture at the right anterior aspect of C1 (arrow). Fracture fragments are seen in the joint space. The odontoid peg is shifted to the left.

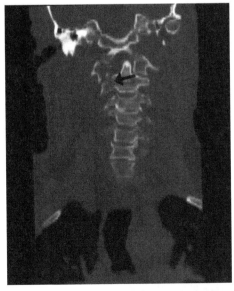

Figure 13.3 Coronal CT reformat shows the C1 fracture as well as a fracture of the right side of the body of C2 (arrow).

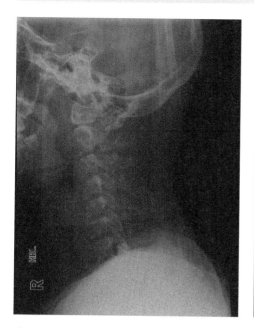

Figure 13.4a Cervical spine radiograph – lateral view.

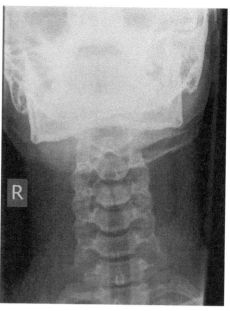

Figure 13.4b Cervical spine radiograph – anteroposterior view.

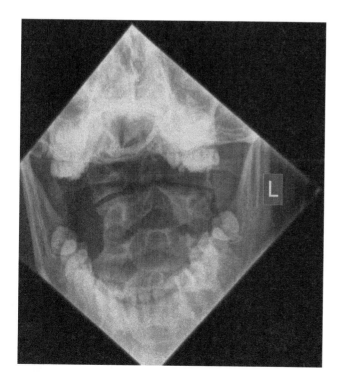

Figure 13.4c Cervical spine radiograph – peg view.

Case 14

A 43-year-old male presents to his general practitioner feeling generally unwell with a history of one stone weight loss over the past month, and more recently a fever. His travels in the last six months have included a trip to see family in India. The general practitioner requests a chest X-ray as part of his investigations.

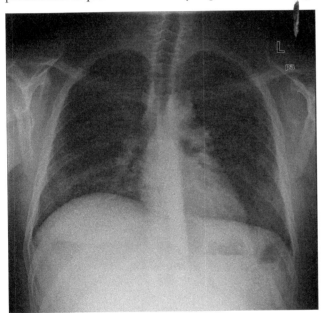

Figure 14.1

Image findings: the radiograph shows extensive tiny nodules measuring ~1–2 mm in diameter throughout both lungs. These are uniformly distributed and equal in size. There are no associated areas of consolidation or pleural effusions.

Diagnosis: miliary TB.

Miliary TB is the result of dissemination of tubercle bacilli via the blood. This means that as well as the lungs, TB granulomas can be found in many organs (commonly the meninges, kidneys, bone marrow and liver). Urgent antituberculous treatment is needed as this form of TB can be fatal without treatment.

It is important to be aware of tuberculosis as it is a disease which is still on the increase both in the UK and worldwide. In particular, the immunocompromised (including those with HIV) are at increased risk.

The first infection with TB is called primary TB which often presents with symptoms of pneumonia, i.e. fever, cough, sputum. The site of primary infection is called the Ghon complex. Post-primary TB represents re-activation of primary infection and this can occur within weeks to many years after the primary infection. Post-primary

TB typically presents with gradual onset of tiredness, weakness, weight loss, fever and cough. Miliary TB can be a consequence of either primary or post-primary TB. TB diagnosis is usually made histologically through the presence of acid fast bacilli.

The differential diagnosis for miliary nodules (defined as diffuse fine nodules measuring <2 mm in diameter) includes:

- miliary TB
- miliary metastases (from cancers such as thyroid, sarcomas, renal cell and breast)
- sarcoid
- pneumoconioses
- hypersensitivity pneumonitis.

Case 15

An 84-year-old male presents to accident and emergency complaining of abdominal pain. He appears cachectic and there is tenderness throughout the upper abdomen on examination. He has a history of pancreatic cancer but cannot remember any more details about his disease. The notes are unavailable and the accident and emergency team perform an abdominal X-ray as part of their investigations.

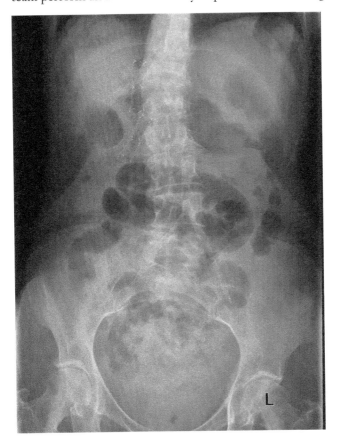

Figure 15.1

Image findings: the abdominal radiograph shows two metal stents in the right upper quadrant. These appear to be lying within the region of the proximal and distal aspect of the common bile duct, with the more superior stent extending into the left hepatic duct, and the more inferior stent into the duodenum. Air can be seen within the intrahepatic biliary tree.

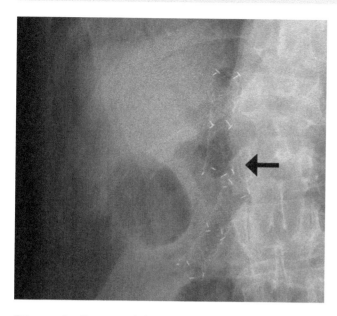

Figure 15.2 Expanded view of the right upper quadrant showing the two biliary stents and air within the biliary tree (arrow).

Diagnosis: Common bile duct (CBD) stents.

Pancreatic cancer typically presents with painless jaundice and weight loss. Cigarette smoking, alcohol excess and DM are recognised risk factors. As in this case, unfortunately pancreatic cancer often presents at a late stage and is inoperable (only 15–20% of patients are suitable for surgery at presentation).[1] Prognosis is poor with only 20% 1-year survival and 4% 5-year survival rates.[1] If the disease is inoperable, then treatment is aimed at palliation. The pancreatic tumour often involves the head of the pancreas where it causes obstruction of the bile ducts and consequently obstructive jaundice (*see* Figures 15.3 and 15.4).

Metallic biliary stents can be placed to relieve this obstruction and aim to prevent episodes of recurrent pancreatitis and a 'closed' bile system developing, which would get infected.

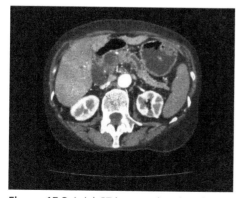

Figure 15.3 Axial CT images showing the dilated common bile duct and pancreatic duct before the stents were inserted.

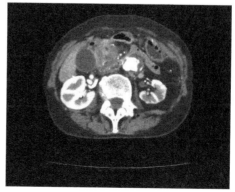

Figure 15.4 Axial CT image shows a large soft tissue tumour mass in the head of the pancreas – 60% of pancreatic cancers occur in the pancreatic head.

Pneumobilia (air in the biliary tree) is usually a consequence of communication between the biliary system and the gastrointestinal tract. The most common cause for pneumobilia is recent endoscopic retrograde cholangiopancreatography (ERCP). Any condition that affects the competence of the sphincter of Oddi, such as a sphincterotomy, inflammation or neoplasm will allow air to reflux from the duodenum into the biliary system. Pneumobilia is also a prominent feature in a gallstone ileus due to the presence of a biliary-enteric fistula formed by a gallstone eroding into the adjacent bowel.

Pneumobilia to the untrained eye can have a similar appearance to portal venous gas. However the two can be distinguished easily by closely examining the distribution pattern of the air. In pneumobilia there are linear branching lucencies centrally within the liver whereas in portal venous gas the lucencies appear more peripheral. Portal venous gas is usually a 'predeath' finding due to small bowel ischaemia and necrosis and is therefore seen in extremely sick patients. Biliary tree gas conversely can be seen in healthy patients.

The causes of pneumobilia are:

- ERCP and sphincterotomy
- surgical and iatrogenic biliary-enteric fistula formation
- peptic ulcer disease
- gallstone erosion
- Crohn's disease
- carcinoma
- emphysematous cholecystitis
- ascending cholangitis.

REFERENCE

1   Cancer Research UK. Statistics and outlook for pancreatic cancer: www.cancerhelp.org.uk/type/pancreatic-cancer/treatment/statistics-and-outlook-for-pancreatic-cancer.

Case 16

A 78-year-old gentleman presented to accident and emergency with a distended abdomen and crampy abdominal pain, getting worse over the last 3–4 days. He had vomited once prior to admission, but his bowels had not been opened for the last three days, and he had not passed flatus for the last 48 hours. On examination his abdomen was generally tender to palpation, and tympanic to percussion. The abdominal X-ray below was performed as part of the subsequent investigations.

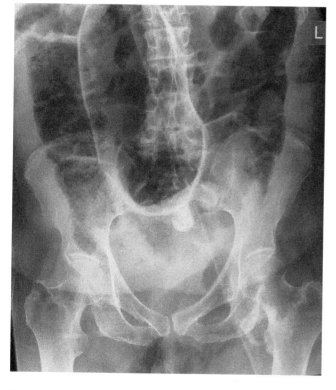

Figure 16.1

Image findings: the abdominal radiograph shows multiple dilated loops of large bowel. In particular one can see dilated caecum/ascending colon to the right of the film and dilated descending colon to the left of the film. No gas is seen in the rectum. Appearances suggest obstruction at the level of the sigmoid (distal large bowel obstruction). There is a large dilated loop of bowel in the centre of the film – this is a loop of rotated sigmoid colon and the diagnosis is sigmoid volvulus.

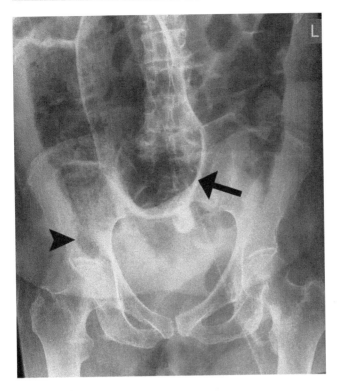

Figure 16.2 Abdominal radiograph showing the dilated sigmoid loop (arrow) and normal position of the caecum (arrowhead) in a patient with sigmoid volvulus.

Diagnosis: sigmoid volvulus.

Sigmoid volvulus is a relatively common cause of large bowel obstruction in the elderly population. The sigmoid colon and its relatively mobile mesentery twist on itself causing severe obstruction. If not identified and corrected, bowel infarction and perforation can occur and the resulting faecal peritonitis is often fatal. Treatment of sigmoid volvulus involves sigmoidoscopy and gentle insertion of a flatus tube through the twisted area and into the obstructed loop – 80% of patients are treated by this conservative management. Recurrence is common (50% in two years).

The commonest causes of large bowel obstruction are:

- tumour
- faecal loading
- volvulus.

Although abdominal X-ray is useful in identifying whether there is large bowel obstruction and whether there is a perforation, it may not always be able to identify the aetiology. Abdominal CT can subsequently identify the underlying cause.

It can sometimes be difficult to differentiate sigmoid from caecal volvulus (*see* Case 17) on the abdominal X-ray, but factors to look for are that the distended loop has an inverted U shape which points into the left iliac fossa, and that the caecum can be seen in its normal position on the right. This is sometimes described as the 'coffee bean' sign.

If the diagnosis is in doubt a single contrast enema is usually confirmatory.

Case 17

A 60-year-old male presents with abdominal pain, distension and vomiting. His bowels have not been opened for two days. On examination his abdomen is distended, tender and tympanic to percussion.

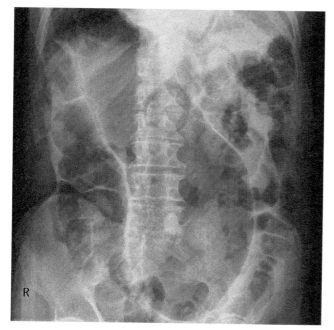

Figure 17.1

Image findings: the abdominal radiograph shows a dilated loop of large bowel within the central abdomen. This forms an inverted U or V shape with the point facing into the right upper quadrant. The transverse, descending and sigmoid colon are collapsed. This is a case of caecal volvulus, where the mobile caecum has 'folded over' into the mid abdomen.

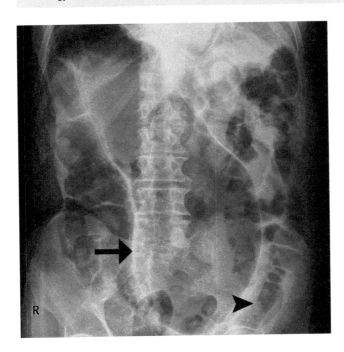

Figure 17.2 Abdominal radiograph demonstrating the position of the caecum (arrow), and collapsed descending colon (arrowhead) in a patient with caecal volvulus.

Diagnosis: caecal volvulus.

Caecal volvulus presents in much the same way as sigmoid volvulus (*see* Case 16), however caecal volvulus is much less common, and tends to occur in a younger age group (40–60 years). The distal large bowel is collapsed in caecal volvulus, and often the small bowel is dilated (though not seen in this case). Endoscopic treatment of caecal volvulus is often unsuccessful and surgery is subsequently required to relieve the obstruction and prevent perforation.

Case 18

A 45-year-old Afro-Caribbean lady has been referred to the respiratory clinic by her GP with increasing shortness of breath and a non-productive cough. She also has multiple raised and tender red lumps on both of her legs below the knees.

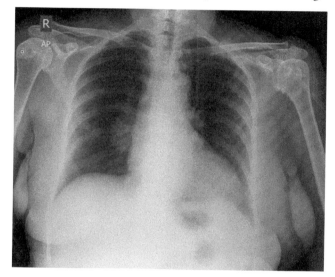

Figure 18.1

Image findings: the chest radiograph shows bilateral hilar enlargement due to hilar lymphadenopathy. Bilateral hilar lymphadenopathy has a number of differential diagnoses including:

- TB
- sarcoid
- lymphoma.

Diagnosis: sarcoidosis.

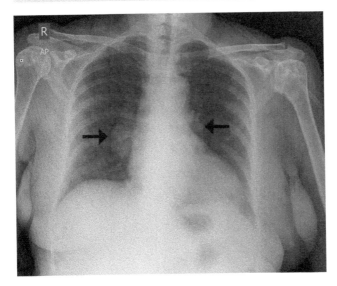

Figure 18.2 Chest radiograph showing bilateral hilar enlargement (arrows).

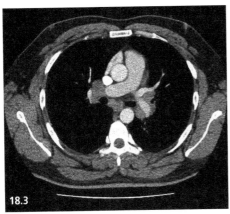
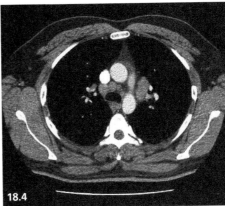

Figures 18.3 and 18.4 Axial CT images showing hilar and mediastinal lymphadenopathy.

Sarcoidosis is a multisystem granulomatous (non-caseating) disease of unknown aetiology. It is seen more commonly in women and people of West African descent.

Erythema nodosum (the skin lesions described in this case) are the commonest presenting complaint, with respiratory symptoms being the next most common symptom. However, in up to a quarter of patients they are asymptomatic with abnormalities incidentally detected on a chest radiograph performed for other reasons.

Overall the lungs are the most commonly affected organ, with 20% of patients going on to develop pulmonary fibrosis. Sarcoid can however affect any organ:

- respiratory system – reticulonodular mid zone shadowing, tracheal/bronchial stenosis, pulmonary nodules
- skin – erythema nodosum
- eyes – uveitis, lacrimal gland enlargement
- cardiac – cardiomyopathy, pericardial effusion
- abdomen – hepatomegaly, splenomegaly, pancreatic mass

- central nervous system (CNS) – cranial/peripheral nerve palsies
- genito-urinary (GU) system – renal stones
- lymphadenopathy.

Mediastinal lymph node enlargement is found in the majority of patients (as in this case). The typical finding is a triad of bilateral symmetrical hilar lymphadenopathy along with right paratracheal lymph node enlargement. The symmetrical nature of the hilar nodes can help to distinguish from TB and lymphoma (in which nodal enlargement is rarely symmetrical).

Angiotensin converting enzyme is elevated in ~70% of patients and levels can be used to monitor disease activity. Diagnosis is usually dependent on histological identification of non-caseating granulomas. Treatment is with steroids.

Case 19

A 40-year-old man presents to accident and emergency with a history of sudden onset of abdominal distension, colicky upper abdominal pain and bilious vomiting. He has had previous abdominal surgery. An abdominal radiograph is requested.

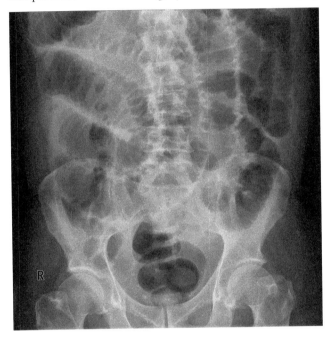

Figure 19.1

Image findings: this X-ray demonstrates the typical findings seen in small bowel obstruction (SBO). There is an abnormal amount of gas in the small bowel. The small bowel loops are grossly dilated measuring >3.5 cm (normal is 2.5 cm) in diameter. The small bowel loops can be identified by the presence of valvulae conniventes. Gas is seen within the rectum.

Diagnosis: small bowel obstruction.

The most common cause for small bowel obstruction is post surgical adhesions, which accounts for almost 75% of cases in the western world. On the plain radiograph it is important to look for signs of a hernia as it is the second most common cause for SBO. A hernia can be diagnosed on the abdominal radiograph by the presence of a dilated small bowel loop pointing directly to or within the inguinal region. Causes of SBO therefore include:

- adhesions
- hernia

- gallstone ileus
- intussusception
- malignancy
- volvulus
- parasitic infection.

Small and large bowel loops can be distinguished by examining the folds. The small bowel is identified on the plain abdominal radiograph by the presence of valvulae conniventes which appear as lines that completely cross the small bowel and the colon by the presence of haustra which only partially cross the large bowel loop. In addition, small bowel loops tend to lie in a central location whereas large bowel loops are seen in the periphery. As well as trying to identify the cause of the obstruction on the X-ray, it is important to look for complications of small bowel obstruction such as perforation which will be evident by the presence of free intraperitoneal air, best seen on an erect chest radiograph as sub-diaphragmatic free air.

The abdominal radiograph is the ideal initial diagnostic investigation as it can often demonstrate the dilated small bowel loops and confirm the diagnosis. A CT is frequently requested to aid the management of the patient as it not only demonstrates the dilated small bowel loops but can also help identify the site and cause of the obstruction, *see* Figures 19.2 and 19.3. It is important to know if the patient has had previous abdominal surgery, as a pathological cause of the small bowel obstruction is highly likely in a virgin abdomen.

The initial management of an acute small bowel obstruction is to pass a nasogastric (NG) tube, rehydrate with intravenous fluids (drip and suck) and correct any electrolyte imbalance. A small bowel obstruction secondary to adhesions can be treated conservatively with the drip and suck method. Surgery is indicated in the presence of strangulation or if conservative management fails.

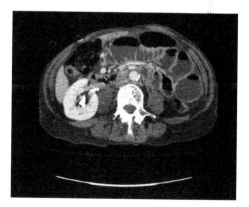

Figure 19.2 Axial CT image.

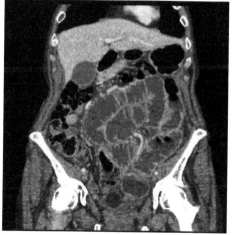

Figure 19.3 A reformatted coronal CT image showing dilated loops of fluid/gas filled small bowel – the underlying cause was identified to be adhesions.

Case 20

A 20-year-old male is brought into accident and emergency after falling off his bicycle. He is complaining of mild tenderness at the left chest wall where he landed on the handle bars, and the CXR below is obtained for further evaluation of the chest.

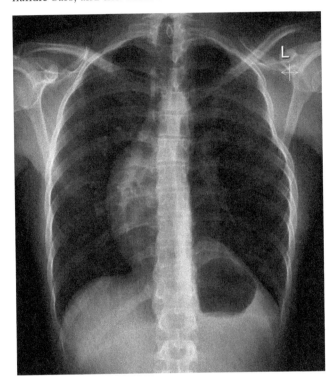

Figure 20.1

Image findings: the chest radiograph shows that the heart is sited on the right side of the chest. This finding should be double checked by ensuring that the side marker is correctly placed (note the L marker over the left shoulder). If old images are available they should also be looked at for confirmation.

Diagnosis: dextrocardia.

Dextrocardia is a congenital abnormality of cardiac position where the heart lies on the right (or more accurately, the cardiac apex points to the right) rather than its normal position on the left.

After identification of Dextrocardia it is important to determine the position of the abdominal organs. If these are also reversed (situs inversus, i.e. the liver is on the left), then the incidence of further structural cardiac abnormalities (congenital heart disease) is only slightly higher than in patients with a normal cardiac position (3–5%

chance). If the abdominal organs are in their normal position (situs solitus, i.e. liver on the right) the incidence of associated congenital heart disease is high (95% chance of congenital heart disease). In this case the gastric bubble remains in a normal position under the left hemidiaphragm.

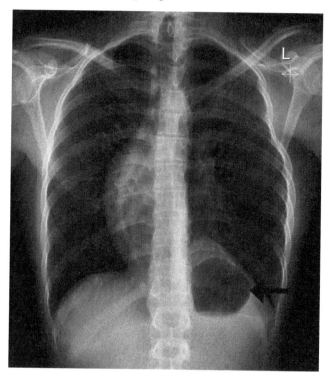

Figure 20.2 The gastric bubble (arrow) is sited in a normal position under the left hemidiaphragm in a patient with dextrocardia.

Dextrocardia can be seen in association with several other syndromes, e.g. Kartagener's syndrome which is characterised by ciliary dysmotility resulting in bronchiectasis, sinusitis and infertility with situs inversus.

Case 21

A 20-year-old man presents to the accident and emergency department following a rugby tackle injury. He complains of left shoulder pain, swelling and has a limited range of movements. He has normal brachial and radial pulses on examination. There is no focal neurological deficit. Radiographs of the left shoulder are obtained.

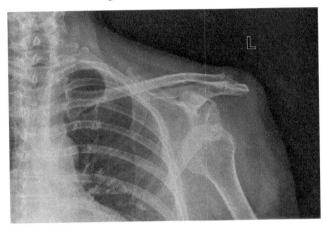

Figure 21.1

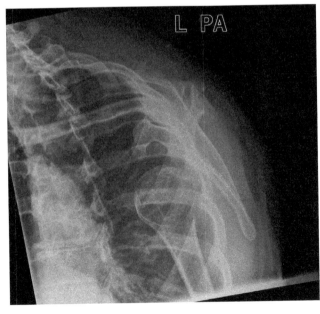

Figure 21.2

Image findings: Figure 21.1 is an anteroposterior projection of the left shoulder. The articular surface of the head of the humerus (H) does not parallel that of the glenoid fossa (G) as it normally should do so, *see* Figure 21.3. Instead, the head of the humerus has slipped medially and downwards and now lies medial to the glenoid (towards the rib cage) and below the coracoid process. This is diagnostic of an anterior dislocation of the left shoulder.

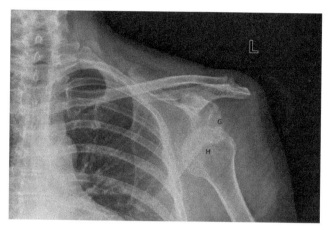

Figure 21.3

Figure 21.2 is a lateral scapular radiograph of the shoulder, also known as a 'Y' view. The 'Y' is formed by the scapular blade (B), coracoid process anteriorly (C) and spine of the acromion (S), *see* Figure 21.4. The glenoid is indicated by the centre of the 'Y' and the humeral head normally lies over this point. In this patient, the humeral head lies anterior to the centre of the 'Y' (overlying the rib cage). This is consistent with an anterior shoulder dislocation.

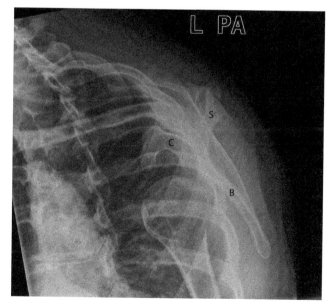

Figure 21.4

Diagnosis: anterior shoulder dislocation.

Glenohumeral dislocation may be classified as either anterior or posterior. Anterior shoulder dislocation is the commonest and accounts for approximately 98% of cases.

The mechanism by which it occurs is external rotation and abduction (usually a fall on an outstretched arm). With anterior dislocation of the shoulder the humeral head is displaced anterior to the glenoid fossa.

When faced with a radiograph of an anterior shoulder dislocation, also scrutinise closely for an associated fracture of the anterior aspect of the inferior rim of the glenoid (Bankart lesion) and for a fracture of the posterolateral surface of the humeral head (Hill-Sachs defect). The Hill-Sachs defect occurs due to impaction of the humeral head against the anterior edge of the glenoid.

It is usually possible to reduce the injury in an emergency department with analgesia and sometimes sedation.

Case 22

A 30-year-old man is brought to the accident and emergency department following an injury to his right leg whilst skiing. He complains of severe pain in his right lower leg and is unable to put any weight on it. He is put into a temporary cast since the initial radiographs are thought to be normal but the doctor is convinced that there is a bony injury. Anteroposterior and lateral follow up radiographs of the right lower limb are obtained.

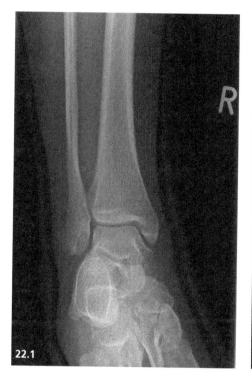 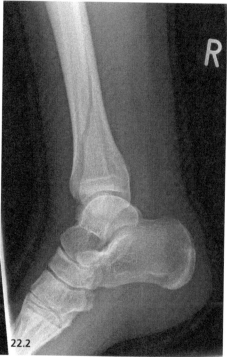

Figures 22.1 and 22.2

Image findings: the AP view appears normal and no definite fracture is seen. However, the lateral view reveals an oblique fracture of the distal fibula. The patient is also wearing a cast.

Diagnosis: ankle fracture.

This case illustrates the general principle in radiology that 'one view is one view too few'. This fracture can be potentially missed if only the AP view is reviewed. Hence, the importance of looking at all imaging available. Preferably the two views obtained should be perpendicular to each other and this rule applies to virtually all radiographs obtained.

As shown in this example, the abnormality may not be visible at all or may be subtle on the first view.

Case 23

A 70-year-old woman presents to accident and emergency after slipping on ice and falling over. She complains of pain and swelling of her left wrist. Posteroanterior and lateral radiographs of her wrist are obtained.

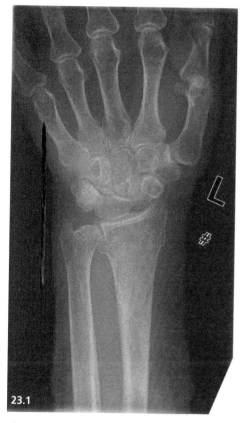

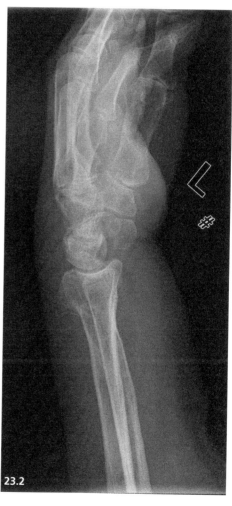

Figures 23.1 and 23.2

Image findings: there is a fracture of the distal radius with dorsal displacement and dorsal angulation of the distal fragment. There is also an avulsion fracture of the ulna styloid process. These features are diagnostic of a Colles fracture.

Diagnosis: Colles fracture.

The Colles fracture is one of the most common fractures of the forearm. It usually results from a fall on an outstretched hand and is more common in adults older than 50 years and in women due to decreasing bone mineral density. The term Colles fracture is sometimes inappropriately used to describe any fracture of the distal radius resulting from a fall on an outstretched hand. However, a Colles fracture describes a fracture of the distal radius with dorsal displacement of the distal fracture fragment. The lateral view is the key to diagnosis showing that the distal radial fragment displaces dorsally. This type of fracture has been described as a clinically apparent 'dinner fork deformity'. Commonly, there is an associated avulsion fracture of the ulna styloid process, as in this example, *see* Figures 23.3 and 23.4.

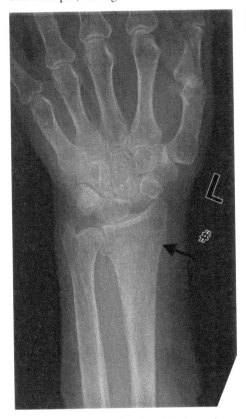 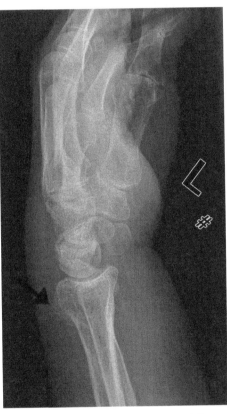

Figure 23.3 Fracture line is visible (arrow).

Figure 23.4 Fracture line is visible and the dorsal angulation (arrow) can be better appreciated on the lateral view.

When the fracture angulates volarly, this is termed a Smith fracture (reverse Colles).

A Colles fracture is usually treated in the emergency department. Following analgesia and sedation the wrist is straightened and is set, put into a 'backslab' plaster and allowed to heal.

Case 24

A 30-year-old man presents to accident and emergency following a fall onto his arm playing basketball. Anteroposterior and lateral views of the elbow are obtained. The lateral view is shown in Figure 24.1.

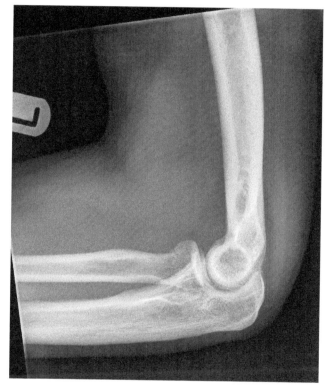

Figure 24.1

Image findings: there is a small oblique fracture of the radial head. The posterior fat pad is visible and the anterior fat pad is elevated and anteriorly displaced. This is termed the 'fat pad' sign and is strongly indicative of the presence of a fracture in the setting of trauma.

Diagnosis: elbow effusion.

Elbow fractures vary with the mechanism of injury and with the age of the patient. In adults, radial head fractures are the most common type and supracondylar fractures occur more commonly in children. Radial head fractures are commonly difficult to identify on radiographs and therefore it is important to look for secondary signs of a fracture, in particular the fat pad sign. Normally there are two pads of fat at the distal humerus in contact with the joint capsule. On a lateral view of the normal elbow, the anterior fat pad is seen as an area of low density (black) along the anterior cortex of the distal humerus. The posterior fat pad is not normally visible.

If there is a joint effusion, the capsule is distended thus displacing the fat pads away from the humerus. The anterior fat pad becomes raised and the posterior fat pad becomes visible, *see* Figure 24.2.

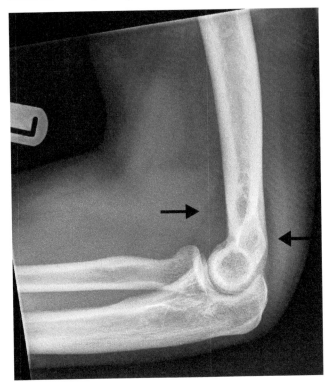

Figure 24.2 Anterior and posterior fat pads (arrows).

In the setting of trauma, the fat pad sign provides a useful diagnostic clue to the presence of a fracture. It is important to realise however, that absence of a visible fat pad does not exclude a fracture as the joint capsule may rupture.

Case 25

A 55-year-old woman from the Indian subcontinent has a chest X-ray performed pre-operatively. She has a chronic cough, but no other respiratory symptoms.

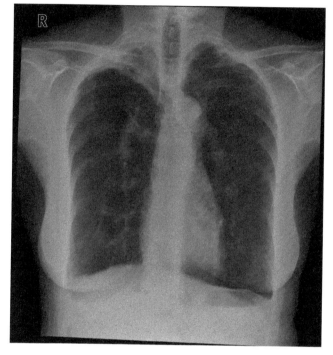

Figure 25.1

Image findings: the chest radiograph reveals irregular linear shadowing bilaterally in the upper zones. Both hila are markedly elevated from their normal positions indicating volume loss in both upper lobes. This is a chest X-ray demonstrating bilateral upper zone fibrosis. There is compensatory hyper-expansion of the lower lobes characterised by reduced lung density in the lower zones and flattening of the diaphragms.

Diagnosis: upper zone fibrosis.

Causes of bilateral upper zone fibrosis include tuberculosis, ankylosing spondylitis, radiation and sarcoid. Other clues to examine for in the chest radiograph are calcification (frequent in tuberculosis), spondylitis (ankylosing spondylitis), evidence of a mastectomy or osteonecrosis of ribs (radiotherapy, e.g. for breast carcinoma) and eggshell calcification of lymph nodes (sarcoid).

Scarring of lung contracts the lung resulting in volume loss as in the case shown. Some of the chest X-ray findings of upper lobe fibrosis can therefore be similar to those seen in lung collapse, which include:

- elevation of the fissures
- tenting of the hemidiaphragm
- elevation of the hila
- tracheal/mediastinal shift.

Fibrosis however will have features of interstitial abnormality with reticular opacities and scarring seen within the lung. These can be better appreciated when the volume loss is less significant.

Clinically these patients present with progressive worsening dyspnoea. On examination they have fine crepitations. Lung function tests show a restrictive pattern. High resolution CT can give a clearer picture of the extent of fibrosis and can point to an underlying cause.

Case 26

An abdominal radiograph was requested on a 50-year-old man who had recently undergone a surgical procedure. This was a routine post surgical follow up film.

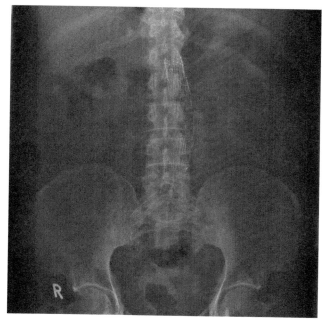

Figure 26.1

Image findings: this patient has undergone an endovascular aneurysm repair (EVAR) which is a procedure performed to repair an aneurysm of the aorta. A stent can be seen in the abdominal aorta extending into both the common iliac arteries. Mural calcification in the wall of the abdominal aortic aneurysm is identified surrounding the lower part of the stent.

Diagnosis: EVAR stent in situ.

EVAR was invented in the early 1990s as a less invasive method of repair of an abdominal aortic aneurysm with the advantages of improved morbidity and mortality. The procedure is usually performed as a combined procedure by an interventional radiologist and a vascular surgeon. Only a select group of aneurysms (~40%) are suitable for EVAR – these require the aneurysm to have a long (>1.5 cm) non-angulated (<60 degrees) neck; be infrarenal in position and be relatively focal. The advantage of this procedure versus an open procedure is that there is a reduced morbidity and mortality. Abdominal X-ray (AXR) follow up is performed to ensure that the stent has been properly deployed and all the parts are open and to ensure that the stent has not slipped.

Atherosclerosis is the most common cause of an abdominal aortic aneurysm with a history of smoking being a significant risk factor. Other causes include trauma, syphilis, infection (mycotic aneurysm), arteritis and hypertension. The abdominal aorta is considered to be aneurysmal if it has a diameter ≥4.5 cm. A normal abdominal aorta usually measures <2 cm.

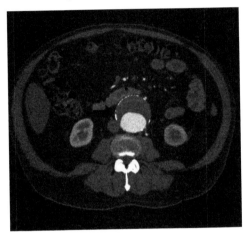

Figure 26.2 Axial CT image of a patient who has had a previous EVAR of an abdominal aortic aneurysm.

In this example the aneurysm is infrarenal which is the most common location (seen in 95% of cases). Other signs of atherosclerosis on the abdominal radiograph include calcification within other vessels, especially the iliac and femoral vessels. Abdominal aortic aneurysms are associated with aneurysms of the common iliac artery in ~90% and occlusion of the inferior mesenteric artery in ~80%.

Abdominal aortic rupture is a life threatening complication of abdominal aortic aneurysm with risk of rupture increasing with aortic diameter. If an aneurysm ruptures then the mortality rate is greater than 95% which is why aneurysms are treated early (surgical intervention is advised when the aneurysm reaches a size of 5 cm) either by aneurysmectomy or an EVAR procedure.

Case 27

The following two chest X-rays are performed on two different patients pre-operatively.

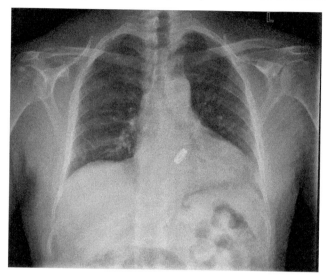

Figure 27.1

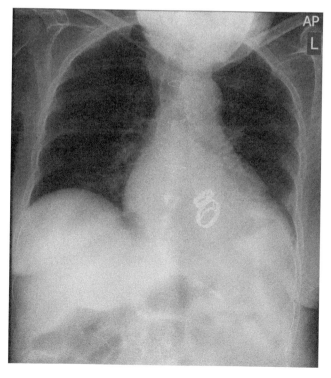

Figure 27.2

Image findings: chest radiographs provide important information regarding cardiac disease. Figure 27.1 shows a mitral valve replacement seen as a high density (bright white) round intra-cardiac device. Figure 27.2 shows two radio-opaque intra-cardiac devices representing mitral and aortic valve replacements. Both chest X-rays show median sternotomy wires and the latter also shows a nasogastric tube in situ.

Diagnosis: artificial cardiac valves.

Mitral valve replacement may be performed for mitral stenosis and mitral regurgitation. Mitral valves are commonly damaged as a consequence of rheumatic heart disease. There are two types of artificial mitral valves – a metal (mechanical) valve or tissue (biological – usually porcine) valve. The disadvantage with mechanical valves is that patients must take anticoagulants for life due to the high risk of thrombosis (blood clotting). The advantage of mechanical valves is their good durability. The risk of thrombosis is less with biological valves, but they have limited durability compared to mechanical valves (12–15 years).

Aortic valve replacement is similarly performed for aortic stenosis and regurgitation. Aortic stenosis is usually as a consequence of degenerative calcification and as it progresses it leads to LV dysfunction. Aortic valve replacement is therefore considered in patients who are symptomatic; patients with a significant pressure gradient across the valve >50 mmHg or valve area <1.0 cm². Aortic regurgitation can occur as a consequence of bacterial endocarditis, aortic dissection, syphilis, rheumatic heart disease or connective tissue disease, e.g. Marfans. Valve function can be assessed using echocardiography and cardiac MRI.

It may be important to correctly identify a prosthetic valve as aortic valves are more susceptible to infective endocarditis and mitral valves to thrombotic complications. A commonly employed method for determining the location of a valve on a postero-anterior chest radiograph is the use of an imaginary line: pass a line from the right cardio-phrenic angle to the inferior aspect of the left hilum. The aortic valve should lie above, and the mitral valve below this line.

The case is shown in Figure 27.2 is a rotated AP film, but the above rule does just about still apply. However mitral valves are usually more vertically orientated and lower down than the aortic valve, which is usually more horizontal and higher up.

Case 28

A 40-year-old man has a chest radiograph taken pre-operatively. He has a slight cough, but is otherwise fit and well with no significant past medical history.

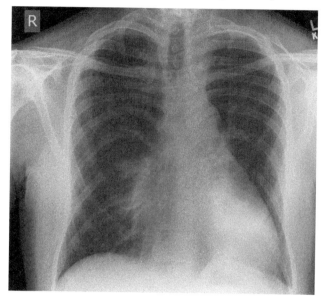

Figure 28.1

Image findings: the chest radiograph shows loss of clarity of the right heart border. In other words, the border is not sharply defined. The anterior portions of the ribs are abnormally vertically orientated and the posterior portions of the ribs are horizontally orientated – giving the ribs an appearance of the number 7. The heart has shifted to the left side of the thorax. This is a chest radiograph in a patent with pectus excavatum (also known as funnel breast).

Diagnosis: pectus excavatum.

Pectus excavatum is a sternal deformity. The sternum is inwardly depressed and the ribs protrude anterior to the sternum. The combination of the depressed soft tissues of the anterior chest wall and the vertically orientated anterior ribs results in loss of the right heart border on chest X-ray, *see* Figure 28.2.

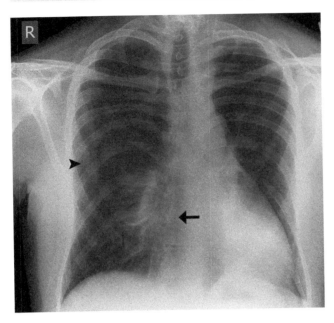

Figure 28.2 Chest radiograph showing poorly defined right heart border (arrow) and vertically orientated ribs (arrowhead) in a patient with pectus excavatum.

This patient also had a CT scan which demonstrates the posterior depression of the sternum and compression of the heart against the spine (*see* Figure 28.3).

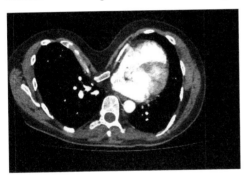

Figure 28.3 Axial CT image showing a significant pectus excavatum deformity.

The chest X-ray findings of pectus excavatum can be mistaken for right middle lobe opacification from, for example, pneumonia or collapse. The diagnosis can be made by looking at a lateral chest radiograph. Thoracic surgeons usually request a CT chest in order to calculate the Haller index. This is the ratio of the horizontal diameter of the chest divided by the smallest anteroposterior diameter of the chest. This is usually <2.5 in normal patients but when >3.25 the pectus excavatum is considered to be severe.

Pectus excavatum is most frequently an isolated anomaly but may be associated with Marfans syndrome, congenital heart disease and other connective tissue disorders. Most patients are asymptomatic, but a systolic murmur can occur from compression of the right ventricular outflow tract. Some patients have mitral valve prolapse.

Case 29

A 60-year-old lady on the intensive care unit has a chest X-ray following a left hemicolectomy and aortic aneurysm repair. She has increasing oxygen requirements and a chest X-ray is obtained.

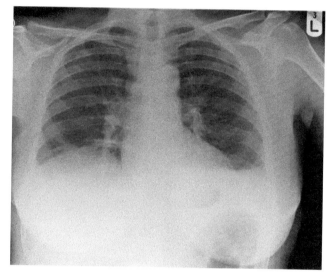

Figure 29.1

Image findings: this chest X-ray was taken in the erect position and demonstrates a moderate sized left-sided pleural effusion. Notice how the upper border of the effusion takes the shape of a meniscus.

Diagnosis: pleural effusion.

The pleural space is a closed cavity between the layers of visceral and parietal pleura. Normally only a small amount of fluid is present in the pleural cavity. Free pleural fluid is heavier than the air and sinks to the base in the upright position. With small amounts of fluid the normally deep posterior and lateral costophrenic angles appear shallow or obliterated. With more fluid, the upper border of the effusion often takes the shape of a meniscus (extends higher medially and laterally). If the effusion is very large, the entire hemithorax may become opaque. Unless there is associated atelectasis on the same side, there may be contralateral shift of the mediastinum. When faced with a chest X-ray with complete 'white out' of one hemithorax one needs to consider three main causes:

1 large pleural effusion
2 collapse of the lung
3 consolidation of the lung.

It is possible to try and differentiate between these by determining whether there has been any shift of the mediastinum. It is easiest to see whether or not the trachea has moved. If there is a large effusion, the trachea is shifted *away* from the white out. If there is complete collapse of the lung, the volume loss results in the trachea being pulled *towards* the white out. If there is consolidation then the trachea will remain central. In Figure 29.2, the trachea is shifted away from the white out consistent with a large effusion. This was confirmed on CT (*see* Figure 29.3).

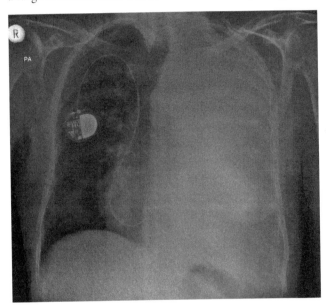

Figure 29.2 Chest radiograph showing a massive left pleural effusion causing white out of the left chest cavity. There is tracheal and mediastinal shift to the right.

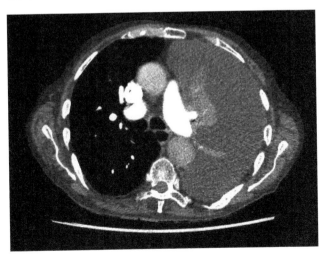

Figure 29.3 Axial CT image confirms a massive left sided pleural effusion as the cause of the white out.

The position of the patient should be considered when assessing a chest X-ray. If the patient is recumbent, then a pleural effusion will layer posteriorly (because of gravity) producing a veil of haziness. Pleural effusions can be divided into transudates and exudates, some common causes of which are listed below.

- Transudate (protein <30 g per litre)
  - cardiac failure
  - hepatic failure
  - nephrotic syndrome.
- Exudate (protein >30 g per litre)
  - infection
  - malignancy
  - collagen vascular disease
  - pancreatitis.

Ultrasound can be useful in the management of pleural effusions since it is the best test to determine if there are any internal septations within the fluid – this is more common with chronic effusions. It can also guide a diagnostic aspiration if there is only a small quantity of fluid.

Case 30

A critically ill 40-year-old man has an NG tube inserted blindly for enteral feeding. The chest radiograph below was obtained post insertion for radiographic confirmation of correct placement prior to use.

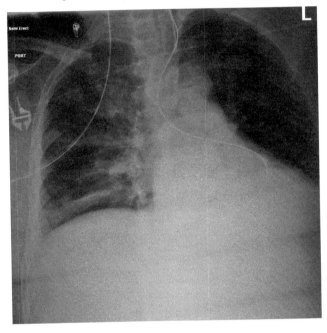

Figure 30.1

Image findings: the tip of the NG tube does not lie beneath the left hemidiaphragm in the stomach as it should do if correctly positioned. Instead, the tube is seen passing down the midline and then deviating to the left side within the chest. The possible explanations for its position are:

1   the tube is coursing down the trachea and left main bronchus with the tip lying in the base of the left lung
2   insertion of the tube has perforated the oesophagus and the tube is lying in the pleural space.

In either case the tube should not be used!

Diagnosis: incorrectly sited NG tube.

Chest X-rays are routinely taken post insertion of NG tubes to verify correct placement in the stomach. The correct position of the tube is beneath the left hemidiaphragm. If the tube is placed in the lung, then complications may arise including pneumothorax, atelectasis, pneumonia and lung abscess.

After the initial chest X-ray, the tube was removed and re-inserted. A further check radiograph was obtained, *see* Figure 30.2.

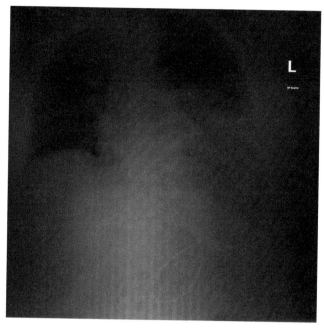

Figure 30.2

The chest X-ray shows that the NG tube lies beneath the left hemidiaphragm, correctly positioned. However, there is new air space opacification in the left lower zone of the lung. The patient's condition had also deteriorated; he had developed a fever and increasing oxygen requirements. A CT scan of the thorax was therefore obtained to further characterise the opacity, *see* Figure 30.3.

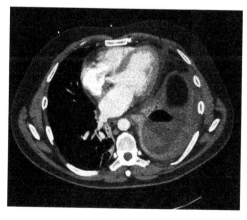

Figure 30.3

Figure 30.3 is an axial contrast enhanced CT of the thorax revealing a rounded thick walled cavity within the left lower lobe. This has an enhancing rim and contains an air-fluid level within it. Appearances are of a lung abscess which had developed at the site where the tube was previously incorrectly positioned.

It is important to get a check radiograph after a line has been inserted to ensure that it is in the correct position. Intravenous central lines need a check radiograph to ensure that position is correct and that no complications such as a pneumothorax have occurred.

Case 31

A 30-year-old man presented to accident and emergency with shortness of breath following a road traffic collision. He was a pedestrian knocked over by a car. On arrival in accident and emergency he complained of chest pain and had difficulty breathing which was getting progressively worse. A portable erect chest radiograph was immediately performed.

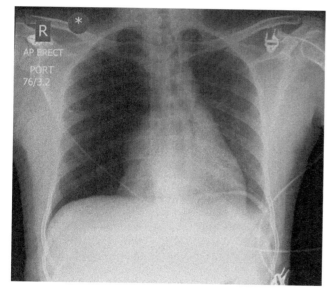

Figure 31.1

Image findings: the chest X-ray demonstrates a right sided tension pneumothorax. The trachea is deviated away from the side under tension with the mediastinum and heart shifted to the left. The right hemithorax is hyperlucent. The visceral pleural line of the right lung is visible with no lung markings seen extending beyond it. The dome of the right hemidiaphragm is flattened.

Diagnosis: tension pneumothorax.

A tension pneumothorax is a medical emergency and should ideally be diagnosed on clinical examination. It is most commonly seen following iatrogenic trauma to the chest in mechanically ventilated patients or following blunt/penetrating trauma to the chest. Other findings on a chest radiograph will include a depressed hemidiaphragm and evidence of trauma such as rib fractures and a haemothorax.

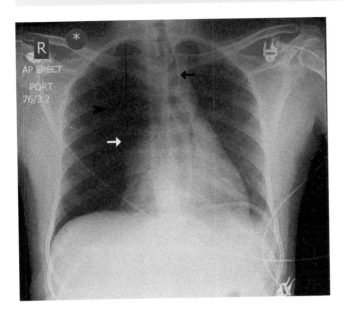

Figure 31.2 Chest radiograph showing a right-sided tension pneumothorax with tracheal shift to the left (arrow). The right lung is hyperlucent (arrowhead). The visceral pleural line of the right lung is visible (white arrow).

A tension pneumothorax is caused by a defect in the pleura that allows air to enter the pleural cavity but not escape. Progressive build-up of pressure in the pleural space displaces the mediastinum to the contralateral side and obstructs venous return to the heart. This results in tachycardia and hypoxia, raised neck veins and reduced BP and if not immediately treated results in cardiac arrest.

Clinical examination reveals absent breath sounds on auscultation, a hyper resonant chest on percussion and contralateral tracheal shift. This is a life threatening condition and imaging should not be performed if suspected as a tension pneumothorax can be rapidly fatal. Immediate decompression of the tension pneumothorax should be performed by inserting a wide-bore intravenous cannula into the second intercostal space of the side under tension in the mid-clavicular line.

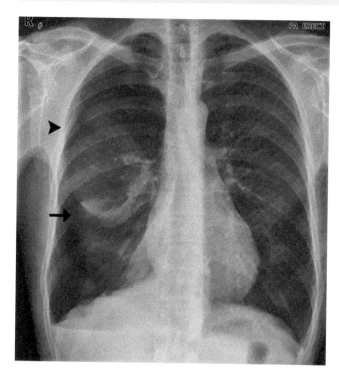

Figure 31.3 Chest radiograph showing a right sided pneumothorax (arrow) with right fifth/sixth rib fractures (arrowhead).

The common causes of a pneumothorax include:

- traumatic
  - ○ blunt/penetrating chest trauma
  - ○ iatrogenic trauma from a tracheostomy, central line placement, percutaneous biopsy or thoracotomy.
- spontaneous pneumothorax
  - ○ primary spontaneous pneumothorax (80%) – apical blebs
  - ○ secondary spontaneous pneumothorax (20%) – asthma, COPD/emphysema, cystic fibrosis, tuberous sclerosis, Langerhans cell histiocytosis, infection, connective tissue disorders and malignancy.

Case 32

A 45-year-old ex-smoker presents to his GP with weight loss and right sided chest pain. A chest radiograph is requested.

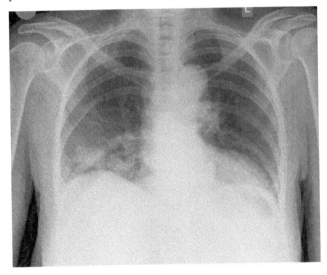

Figure 32.1

Image findings: the chest X-ray shows an ill-defined soft tissue opacity in the right lower zone with destruction of the seventh rib posteriorly. The lateral and the anterior aspect of the rib can be seen. There is also a lucency seen in the inferior aspect of the right posterior sixth rib with cortical destruction which suggests the soft tissue mass is spreading up to erode the undersurface of the rib above.

It is difficult to define the origin of the opacity seen in the right lower zone in this case. The concern from the chest X-ray is that there is an underlying lung tumour here which is eroding through the chest wall and so the patient was urgently referred for a chest CT. CT, *see* Figure 32.2, confirmed an expansile soft tissue lesion arising from the posterior seventh rib with no evidence of direct invasion into the lung. The rib lesion was biopsied and was found to be a plasmacytoma.

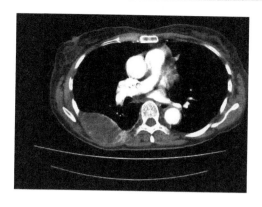

Figure 32.2 Axial CT through the thorax demonstrating a soft tissue lesion arising from the posterior seventh rib due to plasmacytoma.

Diagnosis: plasmacytoma.

Patients with a solitary plasmacytoma almost all progress to multiple myeloma and can precede the onset of this disease by up to 15–20 years. They most commonly affect the vertebral bodies, the pelvis and the ribs. Treatment is with radiotherapy. These patients can progress to show the systemic features of multiple myeloma (which is the commonest primary neoplasm in adults – usually presenting in patients >60 years).

Myeloma is characterised by:

- multiple lytic punched-out lesions seen throughout the skeleton particularly skull and long bones
- proteinuria and renal failure
- hypercalcaemia
- normochromic normocytic anaemia.

Destructive rib lesions can be broadly separated into neoplastic and non-neoplastic lesions. The two most common malignant rib tumours are metastatic deposits and myeloma, which can present as solitary or multiple lytic lesions. Rib destruction can also result from direct invasion from a lung carcinoma. Primary malignant tumours of the ribs in adults are rare with chondrosarcoma being the most common primary rib malignancy followed by osteogenic sarcoma and fibrosarcoma. Osteochondroma is the most common benign neoplasm of the ribs.

Non-neoplastic causes of rib destruction include fibrous dysplasia, aneurysmal bone cysts, histiocytosis X and osteomyelitis.

Case 33

A 53-year-old woman presented two weeks after an upper respiratory tract infection with symptoms of progressively worsening shortness of breath. She had no previous cardiac history and was previously fit and well. On examination she had very quiet heart sounds.

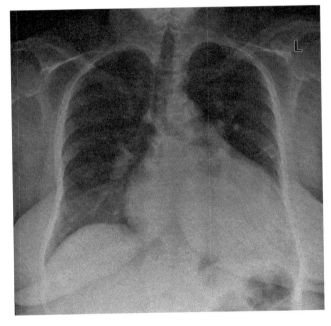

Figure 33.1

Image findings: the heart is significantly enlarged and has a globular appearance. This should raise the suspicion that the cardiomegaly is due to a pericardial effusion.

Diagnosis: pericardial effusion.

Like pleural effusions, pericardial effusions can be divided into transudates and exudates. Causes of these include:

- transudates:
  - cardiac failure
  - hypoalbuminaemia
  - radiotherapy.
- exudates:
  - infection, e.g. TB, viral pericarditis
  - chronic renal failure
  - connective tissue disease, e.g. rheumatoid arthritis (RA), systemic lupus erythematosus (SLE)

- malignant effusion, e.g. due to metastases, mesothelioma.
- haemopericardium:
  - post cardiac surgery
  - trauma
  - post MI, cardiac rupture.

Complications can arise with pericardial effusions when they become so large as to cause compression to the heart. This is called cardiac tamponade. Initially this can present with features of heart failure but can rapidly progress to tachycardia, hypotension, raised jugular venous pressure (JVP) (paradoxically rising with inspiration – Kussmaul's sign) and can lead to cardiac arrest. Echocardiography is a good test to identify the presence of pericardial effusions. Pericardial effusions are usually treated with a drain or a pericardial window.

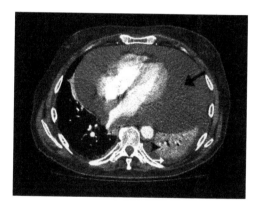

Figure 33.2 Axial CT image showing a large pericardial effusion (arrow). There is collapse of the left lower lobe (arrowhead) due to compression of the bronchus from the massive pericardial effusion. A small posterior pleural effusion can also be seen (white arrow).

Case 34

A 60-year-old man with a history of an increasingly painful left hand was referred for a radiograph by his GP.

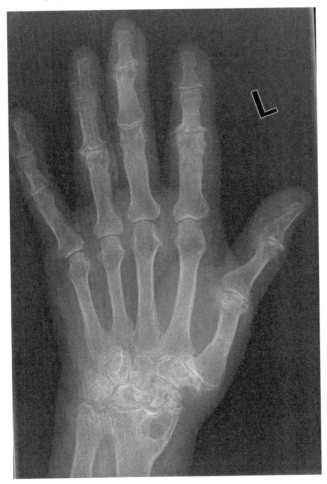

Figure 34.1

Image findings: this X-ray demonstrates the typical radiographic signs found in osteoarthritis of the hand. *See* Figure 34.2 – there is joint space narrowing particularly affecting the carpometacarpal joints, distal and proximal interphalangeal joints and the radiocarpal joint. There is also subchondral bony sclerosis, subchodral cyst formation (arrow) and osteophyte formation (arrowhead) evident on this radiograph.

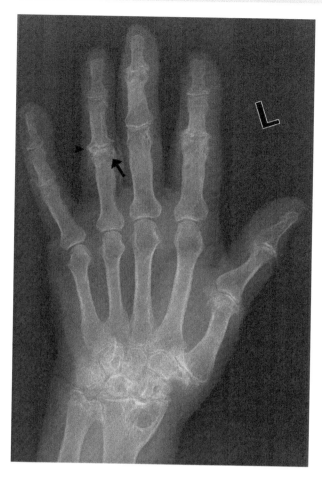

Figure 34.2

Diagnosis: osteoarthritis of the hands.

Osteoarthritis is a degenerative non-inflammatory disease of the joints. Typical radiographic findings in osteoarthritis include localised joint space narrowing, subchondral bone sclerosis, osteophyte formation, bone cysts, subluxation and loose bodies. In the hand, the interphalangeal joints and the metacarpophalangeal joint of the thumb are the most commonly affected joints. Rheumatoid arthritis which is usually the most common differential affects the metacarpophalangeal joints preferentially. Clinically apparent osteophytes in the distal interphalangeal joints are called Heberden's nodes and those in the proximal interphalangeal joints are termed Bouchard's nodes.

Osteoarthritis is categorised into primary and secondary osteoarthritis. If there is no underlying cause found for the osteoarthritis it is termed primary. Secondary osteoarthritis is due to an underlying disease process.

Secondary causes of osteoarthritis:

- trauma – acute and chronic trauma
- systemic, metabolic or endocrine disorder – rheumatoid arthritis, alkaptonuria, Wilson's disease, haemochromatosis, acromegaly, hyperparathyroidism
- crystal deposition disease – calcium pyrophosphate dihydrate deposition disease (CPPD), gout
- neuropathic disorders – tabes dorsalis, diabetes mellitus
- miscellaneous – bone dysplasia.

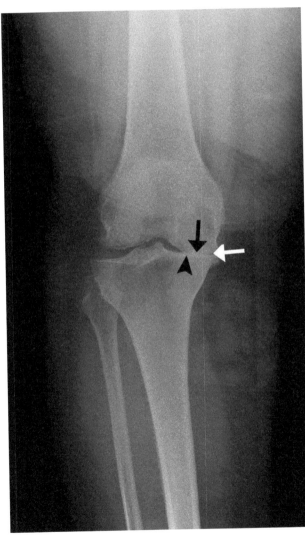

Figure 34.3 Frontal radiograph of the right knee showing narrowing of the joint space (black arrow), subchondral sclerosis (arrowhead) and osteophyte formation (white arrow).

The most commonly affected sites of osteoarthritis are the hips, knees and shoulders.

Case 35

A 52-year-old gentleman presents with a two week history of cough, along with small flecks of haemoptysis. He has been minimally breathless over the last two months. He has a 30 pack a year smoking history. He denies rigors, fever, sweats. His chest radiograph is shown below.

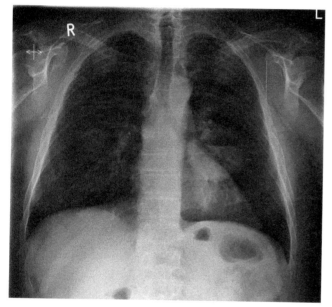

Figure 35.1

Image findings: the chest radiograph shows multiple rounded opacities, some with cavitation. The largest cavity is in the left mid zone, containing an air-fluid level. There are also two soft tissue masses in the apices. There is no cardiomegaly and the hilar and mediastinal contours are normal. This is a chest radiograph of multiple cavitating pulmonary lesions. A CT was performed, *see* Figure 35.2.

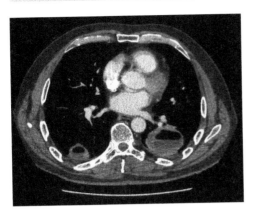

Figure 35.2 Axial CT image showing large cavitating lung nodules with air fluid levels within them.

Diagnosis: multiple cavitating pulmonary lesions.

Cavitating pulmonary lesions can be due to a variety of causes, examples of which are listed below.

- Malignancy:
    - lung cancer (squamous cell carcinomas are more likely to cavitate)
    - lung metastases, e.g. squamous cell carcinoma metastases from the nasopharynx, cervix or oesophagus.
- Infection (pulmonary abscess):
    - staphylococcal aureus
    - gram negative pneumonia
    - mycobacterium tuberculosis. Cavities tend to be thick walled and smooth. They have a predilection for the upper lobes and apical segment of the lower lobes
    - fungal, e.g. aspergillosis.
- Collagen vascular disease:
    - wegener's granulomatosis. Cavities can be transient
    - rheumatoid nodules.
- Vascular disease :
    - pulmonary embolus with infarction
    - septic emboli.
- Granulomatous diseases:
    - Sarcoid.
- Bronchopulmonary disease:
    - infected bulla
    - cystic bronchiectasis.
- Trauma:
    - traumatic lung cyst.

Usually the underlying cause for the nodules can be found with information from the clinical history or examination. When despite this, there is still clinical uncertainty about their aetiology then surgical excision of a nodule for histological analysis is undertaken.

Case 36

An adult male from a psychiatric unit was referred to accident and emergency with a history of sudden onset abdominal pain.

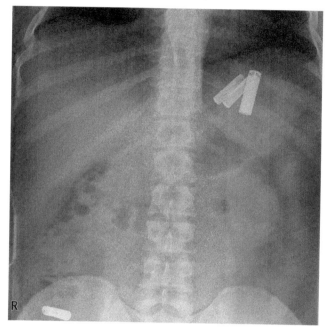

Figure 36.1

Image findings: this abdominal X-ray shows three rectangular radio-opaque objects in the left upper quadrant of the abdomen and one in the right iliac fossa. These objects are in fact AA batteries that the patient has ingested and is the likely cause of the abdominal pain.

Diagnosis: swallowed foreign bodies.

Foreign bodies and metallic artefacts are often seen on the abdominal X-ray. Common foreign bodies ingested include batteries, rings, *see* Figure 36.2 and coins, particularly in the paediatric population. Patients have also been known to present to accident and emergency having inserted and wedged foreign bodies into almost any possible orifice. The management of a foreign body depends on the nature and position of it within the GI tract. The majority of foreign bodies will pass uneventfully through the GI tract. Batteries are important to recognise as they can potentially leak causing erosion and perforation. The ingestion of multiple magnets can also lead to ulceration and perforation, especially when two magnets in separate loops are attracted together. Foreign bodies within the oesophagus and stomach can be easily removed by endoscopy.

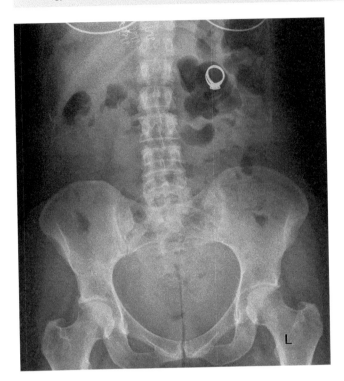

Figure 36.2 Abdominal radiograph revealing an ingested ring.

In this example, the three batteries in the left upper quadrant are most likely to be in the stomach and can be removed by gastroscopy. It is difficult to state definitely the location of the single battery in the right iliac fossa as it lies in the region of the ileocaecal junction and may be in either the distal small bowel or proximal large bowel.

Case 37

This chest X-ray is from a 65-year-old male who had rheumatic fever as a child.

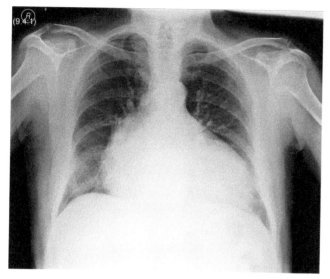

Figure 37.1

Image findings: there is considerable cardiomegaly (enlargement of the heart) with generalised chamber enlargement. The cardiothoracic ratio (CTR) exceeds 50%. There is also mild enlargement of the perihilar vessels denoting mild central pulmonary vascular congestion. There are no pleural effusions.

Diagnosis: cardiomegaly.

The CTR is the maximum transverse diameter of the heart divided by the transverse diameter of the thorax (measured from the inside rib margin) at the widest point. The CTR on a posteroanterior chest radiograph obtained at full inspiration should not exceed 50%. In this case, the CTR exceeded 50% and was in fact measured at 20:29, *see* Figure 37.2.

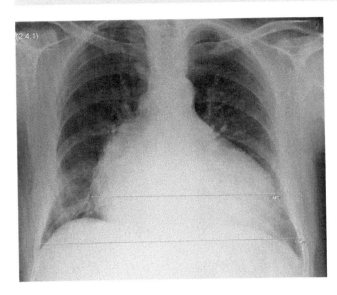

Figure 37.2 Chest radiograph showing cardiomegaly with a cardiothoracic ratio of 20:29.

A small percentage of people will however have a normal heart but a CTR exceeding 50%. It is worth noting that for a neonate, an abnormal CTR is greater than 66%.

Causes of cardiomegaly to consider include:

- congestive cardiac failure (this is a type of ischaemic dilated cardiomyopathy)
- dilated cardiomyopathy – this can have several other causes such as post myocarditis, pregnancy, thyrotoxicosis and alcohol abuse. It is characterised by left ventricular dilatation with global hypokinesia
- pericardial effusion
- valvular disease.

The patient in the case shown had mitral valve disease, severe aortic stenosis and tricuspid regurgitation as a consequence of rheumatic heart disease. Patients who have an enlarged heart on CXR need a full cardiac history and examination to try to identify the underlying cause. Echocardiography is the best first test to look at the heart and can assess LV function, valvular function and determine whether there is a pericardial effusion. Cardiac MRI can supplement the echocardiographic findings.

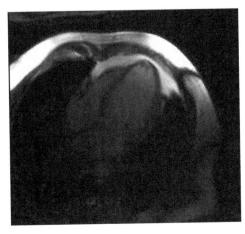

Figure 37.3 Four chamber view cardiac MRI image showing an enlarged left ventricle in a patient with dilated cardiomyopathy secondary to alcohol excess.

Case 38

A teenager presents to accident and emergency having sustained an injury to his little finger while playing cricket. A radiograph of his finger is requested.

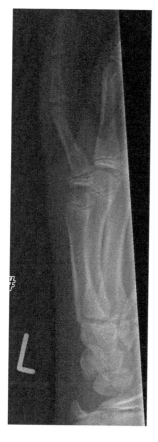

Figure 38.1

Image findings: there is a fracture through the metaphysis of the proximal phalanx extending into the epiphyseal plate. This type of fracture pattern involving the growth plate is classified as a Salter-Harris type 2 injury.

Diagnosis: Salter-Harris Type 2 fracture.

Long bones in a developing skeleton are divided into three parts:

1 diaphysis – the shaft or body of the bone
2 metaphysis – the flared ends of the bone between the diaphysis and the epiphysis. The epiphyseal growth plate is a layer of hyaline cartilage, which is responsible for the increase in the length of the long bones with age

3   epiphysis – these form the ends of the long bones fusing with the metaphysis when the epiphyseal growth plate ossifies.

Epiphyseal fractures which are fractures involving the growth plate are classified according to the Salter-Harris classification. Failure to diagnose an epiphyseal fracture can lead to premature fusion of the growth plate and subsequent limb shortening. The Salter-Harris classification links the radiographic findings to the clinical prognosis with Type 1 fractures having a good prognosis and Type 5 the worse.

Table 38.1 Salter-Harris classification

Salter-Harris classification	
Type 1	Fracture involving the physis only
Type 2	Fracture involving the physis and metaphysis
Type 3	Fracture involving the physis and epiphysis
Type 4	Fracture involving the physis, epiphysis and metaphysis
Type 5	Impaction fracture of the epiphysis

Case 39

A 40-year-old man is brought to accident and emergency following a seizure. When he becomes fully conscious, he complains of left sided shoulder pain. On examination, there is decreased range of movement of his left shoulder. He has normal brachial and radial pulses on examination. There is no focal neurological deficit. Radiographs of his shoulder are obtained, the anteroposterior view of which is shown below. The post reduction film is also shown.

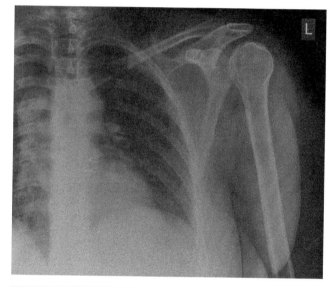

Figure 39.1

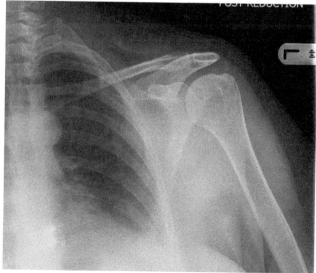

Figure 39.2

Image findings: Figure 39.1 shows the humeral head appearing to lie in the glenoid, however it has an abnormally rounded appearance (like a light bulb). Notice also, the loss of the humeral head/glenoid rim overlap on Figure 39.1 compared to the post reduction film, Figure 39.2. This is a posterior dislocation of the shoulder.

Diagnosis: posterior shoulder dislocation.

Posterior shoulder dislocation occurs as a result of indirect trauma, for example due to a seizure or electrocution. Occasionally it may occur as a result of direct impaction or a fall on an outstretched hand. The normal appearance of the humeral head is not round, but is similar in shape to the head of a walking stick. This appearance is due to the external rotation of the arm when an AP radiograph of the shoulder is obtained. When there is posterior dislocation of the shoulder, the arm is unable to externally rotate fully, giving the rounded appearance. Other radiographic observations which can occur with posterior dislocation of the shoulder include widening of the joint beyond 6 mm and loss of the humeral head/glenoid rim overlap.

Case 40

A chest X-ray is performed on a patient on ITU that is difficult to intubate.

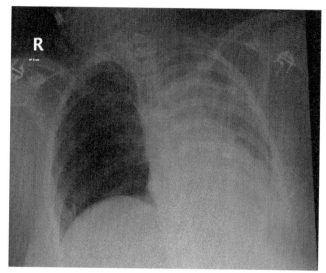

Figure 40.1

Image findings: the endotracheal tube has been positioned incorrectly in the right main bronchus resulting in complete collapse of the left lung. There is also a right internal jugular line in situ with the tip in the right atrium.

Diagnosis: left lung collapse.

This X-ray is an excellent example of the importance of reviewing all support lines, pacemakers, drains and tubes attached to a patient on a radiograph. Check X-rays are often performed to check the position of recently inserted lines such as central lines and NG tubes. It is therefore important to be familiar with the normal position of the common lines on a radiograph in order to be able to detect mal-positioned lines with confidence. Oxygen mask tubing and ECG electrode wires may also often be seen on a chest radiograph.

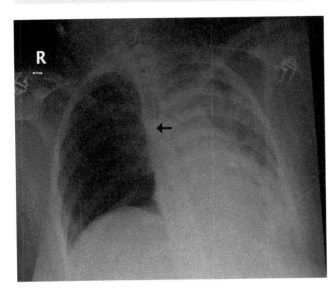

Figure 40.2 Chest radiograph demonstrates the endotracheal tube has been inserted in too far – with its tip lying in the right main bronchus (arrow).

In this example the endotracheal tube has been inserted into the right main bronchus blocking off ventilation to the left main bronchus. The tip of the endotracheal tube should be sited at a level ~2–3 cm above the carina.

Satisfactory positions of common thoracic support lines:

- NG tube – the tip should lie below the hemidiaphragm
- central line – the tip should lie in the distal superior vena cava (SVC)
- endotracheal tube – the tip should be positioned just above the carina
- pacemaker wires – ensure the wires are connected to the pacemaker and insert into a heart chamber
- chest drain – check the tip of the drain lies within the hemithorax.

In this case there is complete collapse of the left lung, so there is haziness across the left chest with some aerated lung in the periphery. There is meditational shift to the left which is demonstrated by the heart being entirely within the left side of the chest. The right heart border is no longer visible to the right of the midline.

Case 41

A 63-year-old woman presents to accident and emergency with severe back pain following a car accident. On initial survey in the emergency department she has no increased tone in her legs; normal sensation and down going plantar reflexes. She is post menopausal and is currently on HRT. She was prescribed bisphosphonates two years previously by her GP which she takes regularly. She is otherwise fit and well. A radiograph of the spine is requested.

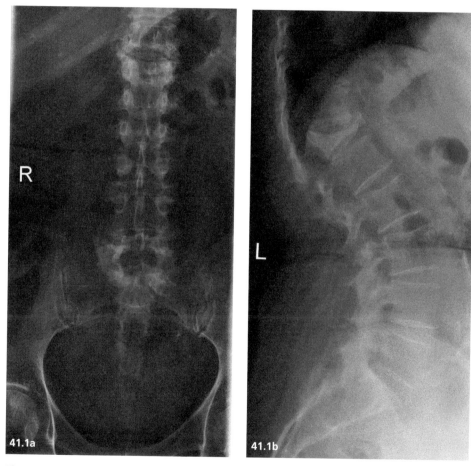

Figures 41.1a, b

Image findings: these images are AP and lateral views of the thoracolumbar spine. The lateral view demonstrates a compression fracture of the anterior part of the vertebral body of T12. The normal posterior concavity of the vertebral body is preserved. The AP view shows an increase in the interpedicular distance at the level of T12, again signifying a fracture of the vertebral body. The paraspinal lines should also be assessed on an AP view of the spine as they may be displaced by an associated paraspinal haematoma. An incidental finding of calcification of the abdominal aorta is noted on the lateral view.

Diagnosis: compression fracture T12.

The standard radiographic views for assessing an injury to the spine are the anteroposterior and lateral views. The vertebral bodies are seen in profile and facet joints are well demonstrated on the lateral view. Vertebral body height and intervertebral disc height as well as fractures of the spinous processes can easily be evaluated on the lateral view.

Compression fractures (also called wedge fractures) result from failure of the anterior column from compressive forces during anterior or lateral flexion. The anteroposterior radiograph (Figure 41.1a) shows buckling of the lateral cortices of the vertebral body as well as reduction in height of the vertebral body. The commonest causes of wedge compression fractures are:

- trauma
- osteoporosis
- metastatic infiltration with a pathological fracture.

A three column spine classification is used to describe injuries of the thoracolumbar spine. The anterior column consists of the anterior two thirds of the vertebral body. The middle column consists of the posterior third of the vertebral body and the posterior longitudinal ligament. The posterior column consists of the posterior portion of the neural arch and adjacent ligaments.

An unstable spinal injury is defined as a fracture that involves two or more columns. It is important to assess the neurological status of all patients following a spinal injury. The spinal cord can be compromised as a result of retropulsion of a bony fragment from the fracture.

Symptoms of spinal cord compression will depend on which level of the cord is involved. If any of these features are present then further investigation with an MRI of the spine is advised. Symptoms will include:

- muscular weakness
- increased tone in the lower limbs
- abnormal sensation in the dermatomes below the level of involvement
- increased reflexes
- cauda equina syndrome – paraparesis, urinary incontinence, saddlelike dermatomal anaesthesia and areflexia.

Other causes for back pain should be looked for on the plain radiographs, especially in the elderly as the back pain may be attributable to an aneurysmal calcified abdominal aorta about to rupture!

Case 42

A 26-year-old man presents to accident and emergency with sudden onset of a headache and vomiting. The headache does not improve with analgesia. His GCS is 14/15. A CT head is requested.

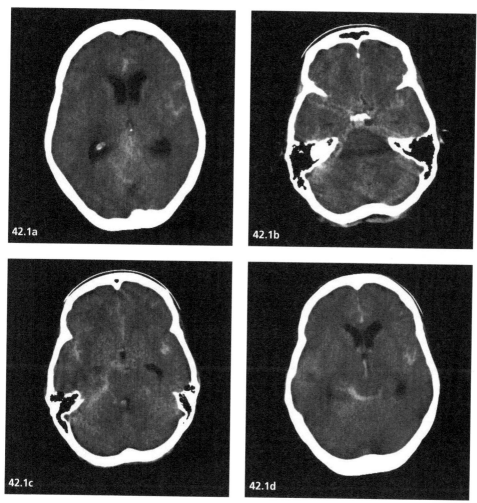

Figures 42.1a, b, c, d

Image findings: four selected images from a CT head show the typical findings seen in a subarachnoid haemorrhage (SAH). There are areas of high attenuation (white) seen in the sylvian fissures, basal cisterns, cortical sulci along the interhemispheric fissure and in the ventricles, *see* Figure 42.2. There is dilatation of the left temporal horn in keeping with early hydrocephalus.

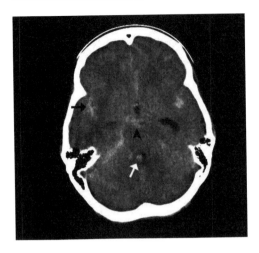

Figure 42.2 Axial CT image of the head shows blood in the sylvian fissures (black arrow) and fourth ventricle (white arrow).

Diagnosis: subarachnoid haemorrhage.

Patients with a SAH present with what they describe as 'the worst headache ever' sometimes followed by loss of consciousness. They have symptoms of meningism with neck stiffness, nausea, vomiting and photophobia. SAHs can occur spontaneously or following trauma. Causes of spontaneous SAH include:

- ruptured aneurysm
- cerebral AV malformation
- hypertensive haemorrhage
- vasculitis.

The most common cause for a spontaneous SAH is a ruptured cerebral artery aneurysm (~70%). The majority of these are congenital with the remainder being due to infection (mycotic) or arteriosclerotic disease. Most of the aneurysms (85%) are related to the circle of Willis with the anterior communicating artery (25%), middle cerebral artery bifurcation (25%) and the posterior communicating artery (20%) being the most common location. Posterior fossa aneurysms account for 15% with the basilar tip being the most common posterior site. When aneurysms rupture they can result in blood in the subarachnoid space; intracerebral blood and bleeding into the cerebral ventricles. Aneurysms can be identified non-invasively by CT or MRI angiography or by conventional invasive angiography. Treatment is either by insertion of coils into the aneurysm to promote thrombosis or by surgical clipping.

A 'berry aneurysm' is a congenital aneurysm associated with adult polycystic kidney disease and Marfans syndrome.

Common reasons for requesting a CT head include severe headaches that are non-responsive to analgesia, significant head injury, decreased GCS and when a stroke (cerebrovascular accident) is suspected. When interpreting a CT scan, it is important to remember that fluid, such as cerebrospinal fluid (CSF), and fat appears as low attenuation (dark). Acute blood on a CT scan is identified as areas of high attenuation (bright). Calcified structures such as bone are also of high attenuation on a CT scan. Basic neuroanatomy is required in order to confidently interpret a CT head.

Case 43

A 45-year-old woman presents to accident and emergency following a generalised tonic-clonic seizure. She has no past history of epilepsy. Her family report that she has been having difficulties with her memory and has been behaving differently recently. There is no recent history of head trauma. The patient is apyrexial with a normal white cell count (WCC) and C-reactive protein(CRP). A CT head scan is requested.

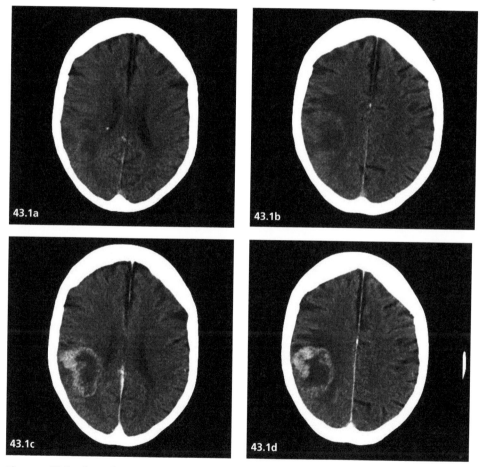

Figures 43.1a, b, c, d

Image findings: there is an intracerebral mass in the right parietal lobe. A region of abnormal low attenuation due to oedema is seen in the right parietal lobe on the uncontrasted CT scan, *see* Figures 43.1a and b. The mass shows rim enhancement following intravenous contrast, *see* Figures 43.1c and d. An MRI has been performed to further characterise the tumour, the MRI image shown is an example of a fluid attenuated inversion recovery (FLAIR) sequence, *see* Figure 43.2.

Diagnosis: primary intracranial glioma.

There are several possible differential diagnoses to consider when faced with a CT scan which shows an intracerebral mass lesion with rim enhancement and surrounding oedema:

- malignancy – primary or secondary tumour
- infection – intracerebral abscess
- resolving intracerebral bleed (3–6 weeks old).

Obviously the clinical history will be very important here, in particular the timescale – infection presents over a period of days; resolving haematoma will have presented with an acute event weeks previously which may be improving and malignancy usually develops over months. Other symptoms and signs are also important – are there any other signs/sources of infection? Does the patient have weight loss or other symptoms to suggest a primary malignancy elsewhere? Further imaging and biopsy can also help to differentiate the cause where there is still confusion.

A patient with an intracranial tumour can present with a wide range of symptoms depending on the size and location of the tumour. Presenting symptoms can include seizures, visual disturbances, personality changes, speech or sensory deficits, ataxia or headaches.

The most common cause of an intracranial malignancy in the adult population is a metastasis, followed by gliomas and then meningiomas. Primary intracranial tumours are more common in the paediatric population. In the adult population, two thirds of lesions are in a supratentorial location whereas in the paediatric population two thirds are infratentorial. Intracranial tumours are classified based on their cell of origin.

In this case the lesion was identified as a glioblastoma multiforme. This is the most common type of primary cerebral tumour and accounts for 1–2% of all malignancies. It is most commonly seen in the elderly aged 60–80 years. They have a very poor prognosis with <50% 3-year survival.

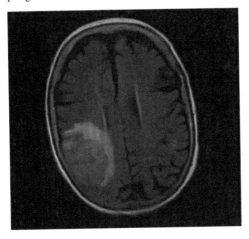

Figure 43.2 Axial FLAIR image of the brain shows a well defined lesion in the right posterior parietal region. The surrounding high signal change represents oedema. A FLAIR sequence is a fluid attenuated sequence so it is T2 weighted but CSF has been made black (usually bright on T2). Any areas that are bright on FLAIR image usually represent abnormal pathology. The periventricular high signal is due to age related small vessel disease (ischaemia).

It is important to assess for secondary effects of an intracranial mass lesion such as midline shift and raised intracranial pressure. The signs of raised intracranial pressure on a CT scan include hydrocephalus, effacement of the sulci and basal cisterns and tentorial herniation. Urgent referral for a neurosurgical opinion should be performed if any of these signs are present.

Case 44

A young woman is seen by her GP with a history of increasing difficulty swallowing and the feeling of a lump in her throat. A chest radiograph is requested.

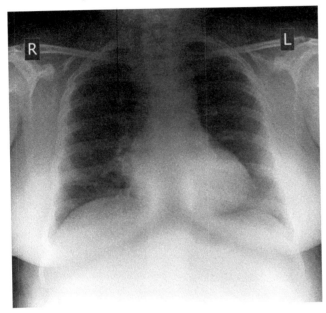

Figure 44.1

Image findings: the trachea is deviated to the right with a soft tissue opacity seen in the lower neck/upper mediastinum due to a superior mediastinal mass, in this case a retrosternal goitre. Surgical staples are visible in the right lateral aspect of the neck due to a previous partial thyroidectomy.

Diagnosis: retrosternal goitre.

There are several causes of a superior mediastinal mass which include the following.

- Thyroid goitre – patients with a goitre can be euthyroid, hypothyroid or hyperthyroid. It is useful to get an idea of the thyroid status from history/examination since this can give a clue to the underlying diagnosis. Thyroid function tests ought also to be performed. Hyperthyroid patients present with weight loss, increased appetite, infertility, tremor, sweating, increased pulse and atrial fibrillation. Hypothyroid patients can present with weight gain, lethargy, depression, sensitivity to the cold, bradycardia, dry skin, slow relaxing reflexes and peripheral oedema. Further investigation includes an ultrasound of the neck to see whether there are multiple nodules or a single thyroid lesion visible – fine needle aspiration (FNA) is performed under ultrasound guidance if there is a single nodule of concern, to exclude a malignancy. When thyroid goitres get very large then they may need to be assessed by CT prior to surgery – this can be useful to determine the degree of retrosternal extension and to see how compressed the trachea has become.

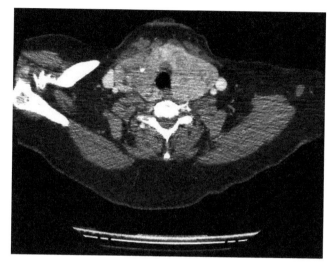

Figure 44.2 Axial CT image demonstrating a large multinodular goitre.

- Thymoma – these can be benign or malignant and can be associated with myasthenia gravis. This is an autoimmune disorder characterised by antibodies to acetylcholine receptors and presents with weakness and fatigability of skeletal muscles.
- Teratoma – these are germ cell tumours which have histological features of ecto/meso/endo dermal tissue so form a mass lesion made up of skin, hair, cysts, bone, muscle, cartilage and teeth; ~10% of these lesions can become malignant and so treatment of these lesions is by complete surgical excision.
- Lymphoma.
- Thoracic aortic aneurysm, or oesophageal mass if large, can also displace the trachea.

The most common causes for tracheal deviation is due to the presence of a pleural effusion, in which case the trachea will be displaced away from the effusion side. Other pulmonary causes of a trachea displaced to the contralateral side include a tension pneumothorax and lung cancer. The trachea is pulled to the ipsilateral side in lung collapse and pulmonary fibrosis. A kyphoscoliosis will also show a deviated trachea on the chest radiograph.

Case 45

A young man has a chest X-ray performed for chest pain. He has a past history of congenital myelomeningocele.

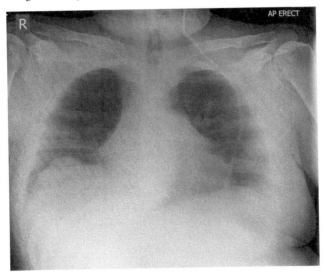

Figure 45.1

Image findings: the chest radiograph shows a catheter coursing from the left side of the neck down the left side of the chest, into the abdomen. The proximal and distal ends of the catheter are not visualised on this chest X-ray. This is a ventriculo-peritoneal shunt.

Diagnosis: ventriculo-peritoneal shunt.

The purpose of a ventriculo-peritoneal shunt is to redirect fluid away from the ventricles of the brain into the peritoneal cavity. It is used to prevent or relieve hydrocephalus (excess build up of CSF within an enlarged ventricular system) which can lead to raised intra-cranial pressure. Raised intra-cranial pressure can lead to injury of the adjacent white matter of the brain and has a high mortality associated with it if untreated.

Hydrocephalus can be communicating or non-communicating. Communicating hydrocephalus is due to blockage of absorption of CSF by arachnoid villi – causes of which can include secondary to subarachnoid haemorrhage, purulent meningitis or metastatic disease to the meninges. Non-communicating hydrocephalus is due to an obstruction to CSF flow within the ventricular system – causes of which include tumours and interventricular haemorrhage. CT brain is useful in identifying the features of hydrocephalus.

The most common type of shunt is ventriculo-peritoneal. The proximal end of the shunt is passed into a ventricle of the brain. This is attached to a one-way flow valve and sometimes a reservoir. The catheter tubing is tunnelled under the skin, behind the ear, down the neck and chest and the distal end lies in the peritoneal cavity. Sometimes the fluid is shunted into the pleural space (ventriculo-pleural shunt) or the heart (ventriculo-atrial shunt). Disconnection or breakage of the shunt may occur, particularly at sites where components are joined or at sites of mechanical stress leading to shunt failure.

Case 46

A 45-year-old man presented to accident and emergency with a five day history of worsening shortness of breath, fever and left sided pleuritic chest pain. On examination there were reduced breath sounds at the left base with a dull percussion note and increased vocal resonance. Bronchial breathing could also be heard at the left base.

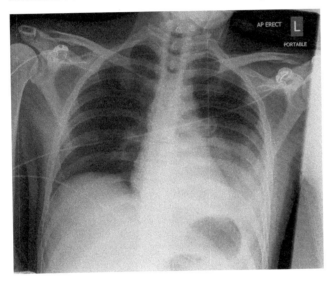

Figure 46.1

Image findings: the chest radiograph shows air space shadowing (consolidation) in the left lower lung zone. The left hemidiaphragm is not clearly seen although the left heart border remains well defined, localising the consolidation to the left lower lobe. The left lung volume is preserved, suggesting that there is no significant associated lung collapse. This appearance is that of left lower lobe pneumonia.

Diagnosis: left lower lobe pneumonia.

Consolidation is due to the replacement of air in the alveoli by fluid or tissue. Fluid can occur for multiple reasons, for example, pus, inflammatory exudates, pulmonary oedema, and blood. Radiographic appearances are non-specific for the cause, however when combined with the clinical picture, the most likely cause can usually be identified. In this example the clinical presentation with fever suggests an infective cause/pneumonia.

Important radiological features of consolidation are that air bronchograms are seen and there is no change in the lung volume.

The differential diagnosis for pulmonary consolidation includes:

- **infective/inflammatory exudates** – community or hospital acquired pneumonia, eospinophilic lung disease, collagen vascular disease (wegener's granulomatosis, SLE), radiation
- **pulmonary oedema** – cardiogenic and non-cardiogenic (nephrogenic, neurogenic, trauma, ARDS)
- **blood** – contusion, pulmonary haemorrhage (Goodpasture's syndrome, bleeding disorders)
- **others** – alveolar proteinosis, sarcoidosis.

The majority of patients admitted with pneumonia will have successful treatment with antibiotics and make a full recovery. In any patient with persistent symptoms, or in an at risk group (e.g. smoker), a routine follow up CXR is advised to ensure that there has been complete resolution of the consolidative change. This should be left at least six weeks however as the improvements in radiological appearance often lag behind clinical improvement. The reason for doing a follow up film is because:

- infection which is recurrent or fails to resolve may be as a consequence of a narrowed or obstructed bronchus due to a central lung cancer. This may reveal itself when the acute episode has resolved
- bronchoalveolar cell carcinoma, a less common type of lung cancer can present as an area of consolidation. Approximately 30% of this type of lung cancer have 'pneumonic' presentation with diffuse consolidation. This will obviously not improve with antibiotics and so persistent consolidation requires further investigation with a CT chest.

Case 47

A 55-year-old man attends his general practitioner feeling unwell with cough, shortness of breath and right sided chest pain. A chest radiograph is obtained.

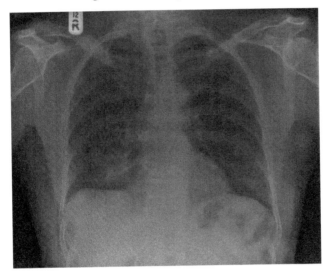

Figure 47.1

Image findings: the chest radiograph shows an ill-defined right heart border and adjacent air space opacification. This patient has a right middle lobe pneumonia. Notice how the right hemidiaphragm is clearly seen, therefore the right lower lobe is unaffected.

Diagnosis: right middle lobe pneumonia.

There are three lobes in the right lung. The oblique fissure separates the upper and middle lobes from the lower lobe. The minor or horizontal fissure separates the middle lobe from the right upper lobe. The right middle lobe is in contact with the greater part of the right heart border therefore disease in the right middle lobe will obliterate this border (*see* Figure 47.2). The silhouette sign, explained on page 13 can be used to explain these findings. Pneumonia (water density) in anatomic contact with the heart (water density) will obliterate that border.

The right lung has three lobes – upper, middle and lower lobes with individual segmental bronchi and segmental arterial branches from the main right pulmonary artery to each of their segments.

- The upper lobe has three segments and consists of: apical, anterior and posterior segments.
- The middle lobe has two segments and consists of: medial and lateral segments.

The lower lobe has five segments and consists of: apical, medial basal, anterior basal, lateral basal and posterior basal segments.

In this case there is airspace opacification within the medial segment of the right middle lobe.

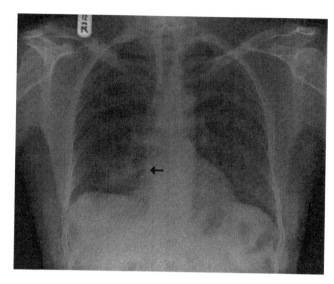

Figure 47.2 Chest radiograph shows poor definition of the right heart border due to right middle lobe consolidation (arrow).

Case 48

A 55-year-old gentleman presenting with a four-month history of epigastric pain, weight loss and haematemesis is referred for a barium meal.

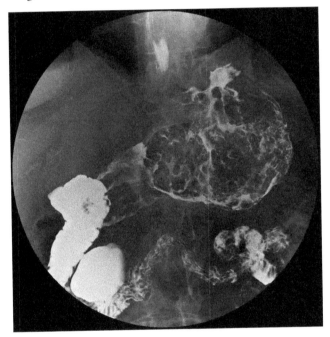

Figure 48.1

Image findings: Figure 48.1 is a double contrast barium meal showing a large polypoid mass within the body of the stomach. The surface of the mass is irregular and nodular with possible ulceration. Overall the appearances are consistent with a large polypoid gastric tumour. Differentials include gastric carcinoma and gastrointestinal stromal tumour (GIST). This in fact proved to be a case of gastric carcinoma. The normal gastric rugae can no longer be seen. (Rugae are folds of gastric mucosa that normally produce ridges when the stomach is distended). Figure 48.2 is an image from a normal barium meal examination with smooth rugae.

Diagnosis: gastric cancer.

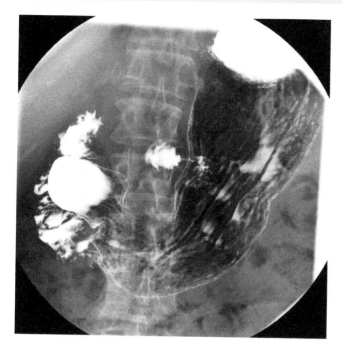

Figure 48.2 Normal barium meal.

Gastric carcinoma often remains asymptomatic until late in the disease. Predisposing factors include Helicobacter pylori infection, pernicious anaemia, atrophic gastritis, smoking and partial gastrectomy. Adenocarcinoma is the most common primary gastric tumour (95%).

A high quality double contrast upper gastrointestinal examination has a role in the diagnosis of gastric carcinoma, along with endoscopy for histological diagnosis. Advanced gastric carcinoma may appear as polypoid, ulcerative or infiltrating lesions, but there is overlap between appearances. Scirrhous gastric carcinoma produces distinctive radiographic appearances.

- **Polypoid** lesions produce a filling defect in the barium pool.
- **Ulcerative** lesions en face may have irregular, scalloped, angular or stellate borders. There may be nodular folds radiating to the edge of the ulcer crater.
- **Infiltrative** lesions are the least common type and can be divided into two types:
    1. scirrhous – diffuse infiltration of the gastric wall by tumour occurs and there is relatively little intraluminal growth. The wall becomes thickened and rigid, hence the term 'linitis plastica' meaning leather bottle
    2. superficial spreading – tumour is confined to the mucosa or submucosa without invasion of the deep muscle layers of the gastric wall. There is nodular thickening or superficial mucosal ulceration. The involved areas are thickened and rigid, and rugae are thickened and distorted.

CT is useful for detecting extraluminal disease, but requires optimal gastric distension. Findings of gastric carcinoma on CT include thickening of the gastric wall, a soft tissue mass and ulceration, *see* Figure 48.3.

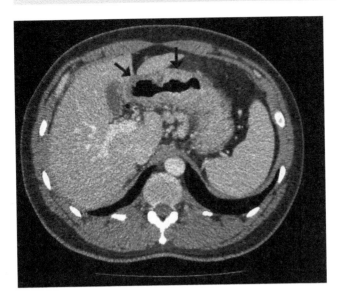

Figure 48.3 Axial contrast enhanced CT revealing diffuse thickening of the wall of the stomach, at the body and antrum, consistent with a gastric carcinoma (arrows).

Case 49

A 70-year-old male presents with dysphagia (difficulty in swallowing), odynophagia (painful swallowing) and weight loss. A barium swallow is requested to rule out an oesophageal lesion.

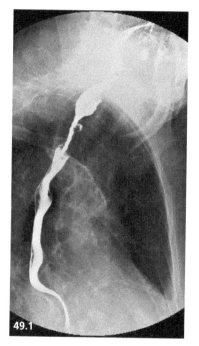

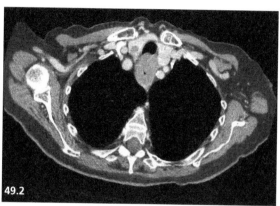

Figures 49.1 and 49.2

Image findings: Figure 49.1 is a selected image from a barium swallow. During a barium swallow, the patient drinks barium, a radio-opaque contrast which appears as white on the radiograph. The barium swallow reveals an irregular stricture of the upper to mid-oesophagus. There is shouldering due to a tumour. This is a malignant stricture due to oesophageal carcinoma.

Figure 49.2 is an axial contrast enhanced CT of the same patient demonstrating circumferential thickening of the wall of the upper oesophagus due to oesophageal carcinoma.

Diagnosis: oesophageal carcinoma.

There are two main histological types of oesophageal carcinoma:

1 squamous cell carcinoma – risk factors include smoking and alcohol
2 adenocarcinoma – this arises in Barrett oesophagus.

Oesophageal squamous cell carcinoma commonly causes an abrupt narrowing (stricture) of the oesophageal lumen by an annular mass. The stricture is irregular. The mucosa may be nodular or ulcerated. Differential diagnoses of long segment strictures include reflux oesophagitis, caustic ingestion, radiation induced stricture and scleroderma.

Barrett oesophagus is a premalignant condition characterised by columnar metaplasia of the distal oesophagus occurring in patients with chronic reflux oesophagitis due to chronic irritation. Characteristically, strictures develop in the midoesophagus and appear as irregular narrowings, similar to that seen in squamous cell carcinoma.

Oesophageal carcinoma may be diagnosed on barium swallow, but diagnosis is best made with endoscopy where biopsies may be taken. CT is performed to stage the tumour (detect distant metastases, for example, to liver and lymph nodes). Endoscopic ultrasound can provide information about tumour invasion and spread to regional lymph nodes.

Case 50

A 70-year-old gentleman presents with weight loss, abdominal pain and new onset of severe constipation and diarrhoea. A barium enema was requested by his general practitioner.

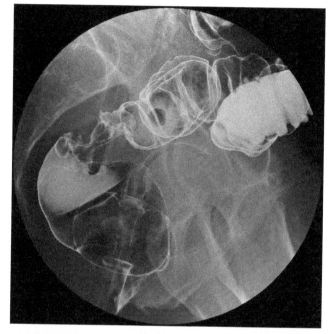

Figure 50.1

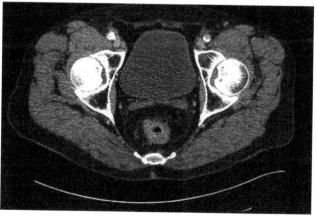

Figure 50.2

Image findings: Figure 50.1 is a selected image from a double contrast barium enema demonstrating marked irregular narrowing of the lumen of the rectum. This is a classic 'apple core' appearance due to rectal carcinoma. Shouldering of the tumour is apparent at the proximal and distal edges.

Figure 50.2 is an axial CT image from the same patient demonstrating circumferential thickening of the wall of the rectum. There is infiltration of the peri-rectal fat.

Diagnosis: rectal carcinoma.

Colorectal carcinoma is the second commonest cause of cancer death in the UK. Presentation can be variable depending on the site of the tumour but symptoms include per-rectal bleeding, altered bowel habit, weight loss and abdominal pain. Patients can also present more acutely with a complication of their tumour, e.g. with obstruction, perforation, haemorrhage or fistula formation.

Colorectal carcinoma most frequently occurs in the rectosigmoid area (~70%). Nearly all colorectal cancers result from malignant transformation of benign adenomatous polyps (the adenoma-carcinoma sequence). Polyps are protrusions from the mucosa and appear as small rounded filling defects on a barium enema (a filling defect is a radio-lucency in a barium pool). Polyps may be broad based (sessile) or on a stalk (pedunculated).

CT often shows a mass or focal circumferential wall thickening. There may be evidence of extension of the tumour beyond the wall, involvement of lymph nodes or distant metastatic spread to the liver, lung and bones.

Treatment is dependent on the staging of disease – CT is used for colon cancer and MRI is used for rectal cancer (*see* Figure 50.3). Staging is by the universally recognised TNM classification. For colorectal cancer, TNM staging is:

- T1 – Tumour confined to mucosa
- T2 – Tumour involves the muscle wall
- T3 – Tumour extends though the wall into surrounding fat
- T4 – Tumour directly invades other organs
- N0-2 indicates the volume of nodal involvement
- M0-1 indicates whether or not there is metastatic disease.

If disease is confined to colon/rectum then it can be treated surgically. If there is diffuse metastasic disease then chemotherapy is used. Sometimes chemotherapy is used to downstage locally advanced disease to then allow for a surgical resection.

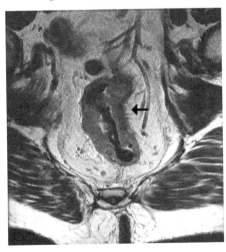

Figure 50.3 Axial T2 weighted MRI image of the rectum shows circumferential thickening of the rectal wall with streaky extension of tumour through the left wall into the perirectal fat (arrow).

Case 51

A 60-year-old lady presents to her GP with a change in bowel habit. She occasionally has some abdominal pain and denies rectal bleeding. She has a background history of constipation. She is referred for a double contrast barium enema to rule out a colonic lesion.

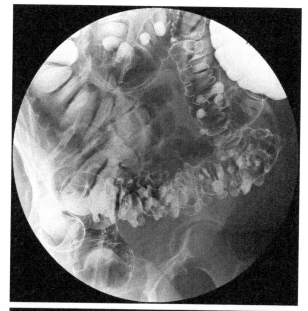

Figure 51.1

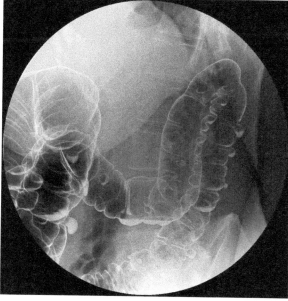

Figure 51.2

Image findings: Figure 51.1 and Figure 51.2 are two different views from a double contrast barium enema. There are multiple barium filled saccular out-pouchings from the colon which represent colonic diverticula. The changes are most severe in the sigmoid (*see* Figure 51.1) and this patient has diverticular disease of the colon.

Diagnosis: diverticular disease of the colon.

A barium enema is performed by inserting a tube into the rectum. Barium (a radio-opaque contrast medium which shows as white) is introduced through the tube into the colon to coat the mucosal lining. Air is also introduced through the tube into the colon in order to provide better mucosal detail (hence, 'double contrast').

Diverticular disease on a barium enema shows as flask or sac like out-pouchings outside the colonic lumen. En face (the surface presented to view), they may be seen as ring shadows or round barium collections. It is often very difficult to differentiate between a diverticulum and a polyp.

Diverticular disease is a condition of the Western world, thought to be related to a low fibre diet and diet of processed food. The condition becomes more common with age. Diverticula develop in the bowel at natural areas of weakness where blood vessels enter the bowel wall. They are acquired herniations of mucosa and submucosa through the muscular layers of the bowel. Chronic disease results in muscular thickening of the colonic wall.

Complications of diverticular disease include:

- diverticulitis (inflammation of diverticula) which can lead to perforation or peri-colic abscess formation. Treatment is by antibiotics with interventional radiological/surgical intervention if there is a large abscess present
- fistula formation – if the diverticulae become inflamed and stick to the bladder then a fistula can develop. This leads to pneumaturia and recurrent urinary tract infections. Fistula to the vagina or small bowel can also occur. Fistuale require surgical repair, *see* Figures 51.3 and 51.4
- bleeding can also occur.

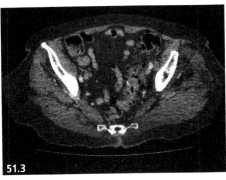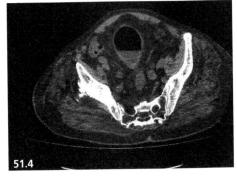

Figures 51.3 and 51.4 Axial CT images show multiple small diverticuli with fistulation to the bladder – an air/fluid level is seen within the bladder.

Case 52

A 60-year-old gentleman presents with progressive dysphagia. His symptoms appear to get worse through the meal till he gets almost complete dysphagia by the end of the meal. A barium swallow is requested to assess the pharynx and oesophagus.

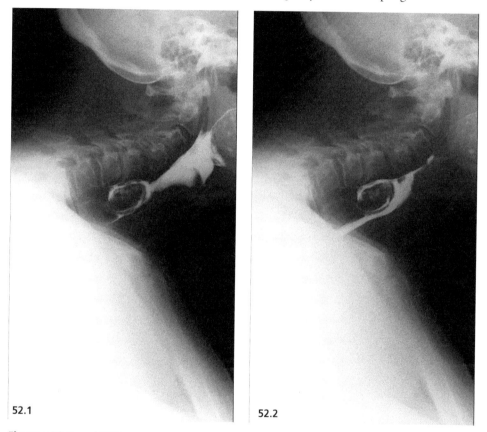

52.1

52.2

Figures 52.1 and 52.2

Image findings: Figures 52.1 and Figure 52.2 are selected images obtained during a barium swallow which reveals a rounded sac posterior to and connected to the oesophagus. There is a residual pool of contrast (white) in the pouch. Contrast is seen to flow past the sac and through the oesophagus as demonstrated in Figure 52.2. This is a pharyngeal pouch.

Diagnosis: pharyngeal pouch.

A pharyngeal pouch, also known as a Zenker diverticulum is an outpouching of the posterior hypopharynx. It arises from the posterior pharyngeal wall just above the level of C5/C6 disk. The diverticulum extends inferiorly and usually to the left side of the oesophagus. It may grow to a variable size but can reach many centimetres in size. Patients may complain of upper dysphagia (as the distended sac compresses the oesophagus), regurgitation of food, cough, halitosis and gurgling noises when swallowing. It usually occurs in older adult males.

The pharynx extends from the base of the skull to the lower border of the cricoid cartilage, where it becomes continuous with the oesophagus. It is divided into the nasopharynx, oropharynx and laryngopharynx. The nasopharynx extends from the skull base to the soft palate. The oropharynx extends from the soft palate to the hyoid bone. The laryngopharynx extends from the hyoid bone to the cricopharyngeus muscle. The outer muscle layer of the pharynx consists of the superior, middle and inferior constrictors. The inferior constrictor which forms the posterior and lateral walls of the laryngopharynx consists of the thyropharyngeus and cricopharyngeus. Between these muscles is a potentially weak area (Killian's dehiscence) through which a pharyngeal pouch may develop.

Complications of a pharyngeal pouch include aspiration pneumonia as the food may accumulate in the pouch and subsequently be regurgitated and aspirated. There is also a small risk of squamous cell carcinoma. The pouch may be surgically treated if large and symptomatic.

Case 53

A 60-year-old lady who underwent surgery for a fractured neck of femur 12 days previously complains of a sudden onset of dyspnoea, cough and pleuritic chest pain.

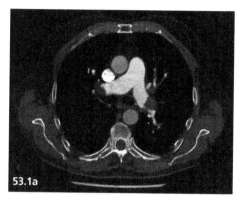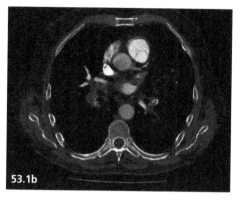

Figures 53.1a, b

Image findings: Figures 53.1a and b are from a CT pulmonary angiography (CTPA). In this technique, intravenous contrast is injected via a vein in the arm and the thorax is scanned when the concentration of contrast is highest in the pulmonary arteries. The aim is to give optimal opacification of the pulmonary vessels so that filling defects can be easily identified. Contrast is seen as white areas in the arteries.

This CTPA reveals multiple filling defects in the left and right main pulmonary arteries (*see* Figure 53.1a) and also the lobar arteries (*see* Figure 53.1b).

Diagnosis: pulmonary embolism.

Pulmonary embolism (PE) is the occlusion of a pulmonary artery or one its branches, usually due to embolisation of a thrombus from deep veins of the leg. Risk factors for PE include immobility (hospitalised, post-operative), pregnancy, hypercoaguable states and malignancy. Diagnosis is made by a combination of clinical findings together with imaging and laboratory tests such as D-dimer.

Chest radiography should be obtained in all patients suspected of pulmonary embolism (PE). Its main purpose is to exclude common conditions that may be attributable to the patient's symptoms such as a pneumonia or pneumothorax. The radiographic changes of PE include:

* oligaemia – this is a decrease in the size or number of vessels due to vascular obstruction, with or without distended proximal vessels. This is known as Westermark sign
* linear atelectasis and peripheral air space opacification
* changes suggesting volume loss, e.g. diaphragmatic elevation

- pleural effusion
- Hampton's hump – this is a pleural based wedge-shaped opacity with a rounded convex apex toward the hilum due to an infarct. However, most cases of pulmonary embolism do not result in lung infarction
- enlargement of the right side of the heart (uncommon).

However, it is important to remember that the chest radiograph is normal in a significant number of patients. Figure 53.2 is the chest X-ray obtained for this patient which is normal.

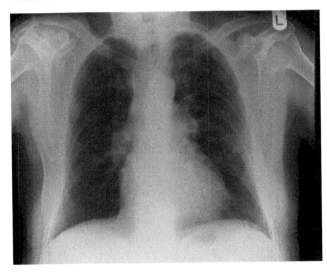

Figure 53.2 It is not unusual for a patient with a pulmonary embolus to have a normal chest radiograph.

Plasma D-dimer is a sensitive but non-specific indicator of the presence of venous thrombosis (sensitivity of 98%–100%). This means that if the D-dimer test is *negative* then the patient almost certainly *does not* have a PE. If the test is *positive* then the patient *may* have a PE (the test is non-specific so can also be positive in patients who have infection or have had recent surgery/trauma). When used with risk stratification algorithms – clinical history combined with a D-dimer is very good at identifying which patients need further investigation. Patients who have a low or intermediate clinical risk of having a PE should have a D-dimer first and if negative, PE is excluded and if positive then they need a further test, e.g. CTPA. If the risk of having a PE is high then this group should progress straight to having a CTPA.

Ventilation/perfusion lung scintigraphy has a role in the investigation of pulmonary embolism if the chest X-ray is normal. CTPA is now used as the 'gold standard' in the investigation of suspected PE.

CTPA also allows assessment of the main pulmonary artery and the right ventricle. Significant pulmonary emboli have a poor morbidity and mortality – CT allows for assessment of the main pulmonary artery (this is dilated if measures >2.9 cm – a sign of pulmonary artery hypertension) and also the right ventricle (a ratio of RV/LV diameter of >1.5 is considered a poor prognostic sign).

Case 54

A 50-year-old woman has a routine chest X-ray taken pre-operatively. She currently has no respiratory symptoms.

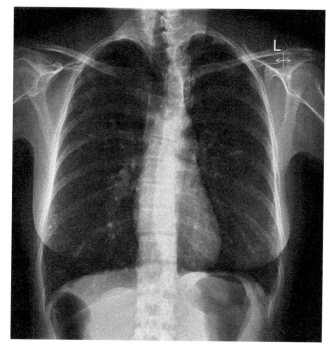

Figure 54.1

Image findings: Figure 54.1 is a frontal chest radiograph revealing multiple diffuse small calcified (white) nodules. This is a patient with healed chicken pox pneumonia.

Diagnosis: chicken pox pneumonia.

Chicken pox is caused by herpes varicella zoster virus. It is a common infection of childhood and usually follows a benign course. Infection in adults occurs less frequently and occurs mostly in the third to fifth decade. Varicella pneumonia is the most common complication and is more severe as an adult infection. Wheezing and tachypnoea 3–4 days after the appearance of a rash typically occurs. Immunocompromised individuals or with lymphoma are at risk. Varicella pneumonia can progress to fulminant respiratory failure. Treatment is with acyclovir.

After resolution of infection, chest radiographs typically reveal small nodular opacities 5mm in diameter scattered diffusely in both lungs. These opacities usually completely resolve, but may subsequently calcify to produce innumerable small (2 to 3 mm) calcified nodules.

There are many causes of small dense nodules on a chest X-ray:

- tuberculosis
- silicosis
- metastases (osteosarcoma, chondrosarcoma, adenocarcinoma of the colon or breast and ovarian carcinoma).

In chicken pox pneumonia, review of previous chest radiographs will show that these lesions are stable and long standing.

Case 55

A young woman has a chest radiograph performed following a procedure done in the interventional radiology suite. She presented a few days earlier with epistaxis, dyspnoea and haemoptysis. She was noted to have superficial small red vascular blemishes (telangiectasis) on initial clinical examination.

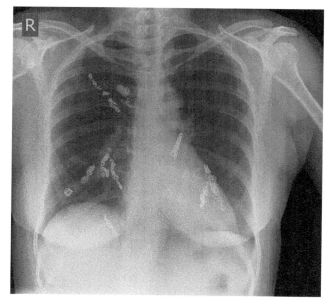

Figure 55.1

Image findings: this is a PA chest radiograph of a patient with multiple arteriovenous malformations (AVMs) that have been treated with coil embolisation.

Diagnosis: multiple pulmonary arteriovenous malformations treated with coil embolisation.

A pulmonary AVM represents an abnormal vascular communication between a pulmonary artery and vein or a systemic artery and pulmonary vein. It is commonly seen in hereditary haemorrhagic telangiectasia (HHT), a condition also known as Rendu-Osler-Weber syndrome. Approximately 70% of patients with a pulmonary AVM will have Rendu-Osler-Weber disease whereas only 15% of patients with the disease will have pulmonary AVMs.

Rendu-Osler-Weber syndrome is an autosomal dominant inherited disorder characterised by multiple telangiectasia which can present as recurrent epistaxis, shortness of breath, recurrent GI bleeding, subarachnoid haemorrhage and haemoptysis.

Pulmonary AVMs are commonly found in the lower lobes of the lungs and appear as sharply defined oval/round masses of varying sizes. A pulmonary AVM is a differential diagnosis for a solitary pulmonary nodule on a chest radiograph. Multiple pulmonary AVMs are seen in up to a third of individuals. A pulmonary angiogram is the gold standard investigation for the detection of a pulmonary AVM, however it is now usual practice to make the initial diagnosis with a contrasted CT chest scan. A CT will accurately define the anatomy and demonstrate the vascular mass along with the enlarged feeding arteries and draining veins.

The procedure of choice for the management of pulmonary AVMs is therapeutic embolisation of the feeding arteries by an interventional radiologist. A pulmonary angiogram is performed by inserting a catheter into the pulmonary artery to locate the arteriovenous malformation. Embolisation is then performed using coils, as in this case, or detachable balloons to occlude the feeding arteries. Lung surgery is reserved for large pulmonary AVMs or when interventional embolisation is contraindicated.

Case 56

A 43-year-old woman was readmitted to hospital a week after having elective laparoscopic cholecystectomy. She was complaining of right upper quadrant pain and had a fever. She had raised WCC and a raised CRP. She also had some shortness of breath which had been getting worse over the last four days. A chest radiograph was requested.

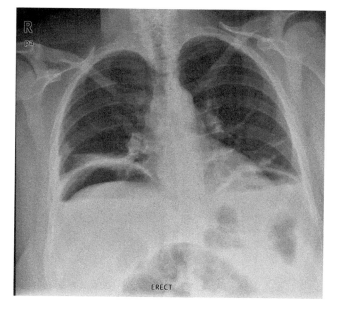

Figure 56.1

Image findings: the chest radiograph shows an air fluid level under the right hemidiaphragm. There was concern that the patient had a perforated intraabdominal viscus and therefore an urgent CT chest was requested, *see* Figure 56.2. The axial CT chest examination shows a large collection under the diaphragm with an air fluid level within it. This is displacing the liver medially and inferiorly away from it. Appearances here are of a subphrenic abscess.

Diagnosis: subphrenic abscess.

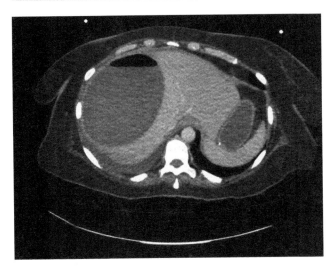

Figure 56.2

A subphrenic abscess is an infected fluid collection between the diaphragm and the liver. The free air under the diaphragm is actually air within the abscess cavity. The cavity can fill with pus which makes radiological diagnosis much harder. There are however usually other signs – elevation of the hemidiaphragm; lower lobe collapse/consolidation, pleural effusion due to localised inflammation. Subphrenic abscesses are easily identified with ultrasound or CT and these can also be used to guide insertion of a drain, *see* Figure 56.3.

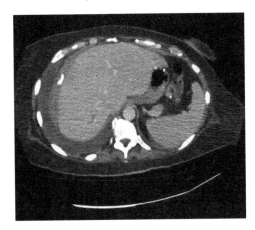

Figure 56.3 Axial CT image of the upper abdomen shows a drain in the remnant of the abscess collection which has now almost completely resolved. Note that even though on Figure 56.2 the collection may appear to lie within the liver, the liver is in fact completely normal on the post drainage film. The abscess has a rounded shape and was pushing the liver medially and inferiorly away.

Case 57

A 40-year-old woman visits her GP with a history of right upper quadrant pain and nausea which is exacerbated by fatty foods. The GP requests an ultrasound of the abdomen to investigate further.

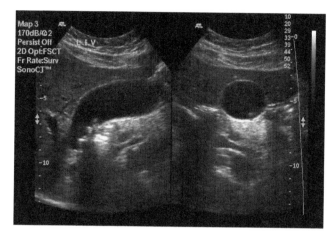

Figure 57.1

Image findings: the ultrasound image demonstrates a few small calculi (stones) within the gallbladder. The gallbladder calculi appear echogenic (bright) with posterior acoustic shadowing.

Diagnosis: gallbladder calculi.

Ultrasound is the modality of choice for the initial investigation of abdominal pain. The liver, gallbladder, biliary tree, pancreas, spleen, kidneys and bladder can all be visualised and assessed. The prevalence of gallbladder stones in the population is approximately 15%, however, only 15%–20% of patients with gallstones will be symptomatic. The majority (80%) of gallstones are composed of cholesterol with the remainder being black pigment stones composed of calcium bilirubinate. However, 15% of gallstones will be sufficiently calcified to be visible on an abdominal radiograph, *see* Figure 57.2.

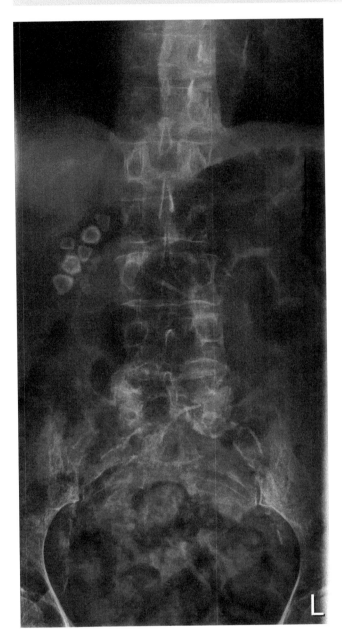

Figure 57.2 Abdominal radiograph showing rounded calcified gallstones in the right upper quadrant.

On ultrasound, gallbladder stones appear as echogenic foci with posterior acoustic shadowing as demonstrated in this case. In acute cholecystitis, additional findings such as oedematous thickening of the gallbladder wall and pericholecystic fluid may be present. Intra- and extra- hepatic biliary dilatation may also be evident on ultrasound if there is biliary obstruction due to a stone.

Ultrasound can confirm the presence of gallstones in the gallbladder, cystic duct or common bile duct. It will also assess for dilatation of the common bile duct secondary to a stone which may be causing an obstructive jaundice. The patient's symptoms will differ depending on the site of the stone and whether there is associated inflammation or infection. Cholecystitis is usually managed with antibiotics acutely with a definitive laparoscopic cholecystectomy performed electively. If there is bile duct dilatation on ultrasound, magnetic resonance cholangiopancreatography (MRCP) may be performed to visualise the anatomy of the biliary tree and assess for any biliary stones or other biliary pathology. Figures 57.3 a and b are images taken from a MRCP study showing multiple small filling defects consistent with small stones.

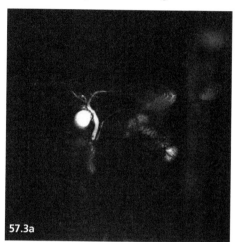 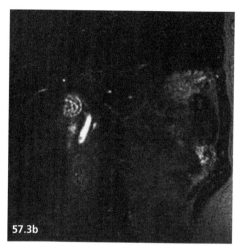

Figures 57.3a, b Selected images from an MRCP study demonstrating multiple stones in the gallbladder and a solitary stone in the distal common bile duct.

If gallstones are present in the bile duct, an ERCP would then be performed to remove the stone in the bile duct prior to a cholecystectomy.

Case 58

A young man attending the emergency department following blunt trauma to his chest in a road traffic collision complains of right-sided chest pain and dyspnoea. He was the driver of the car and his chest hit the steering wheel after a head on collision with another car. Initial CXR showed a right pneumothorax and a chest drain was inserted. An erect follow-up chest X-ray is obtained.

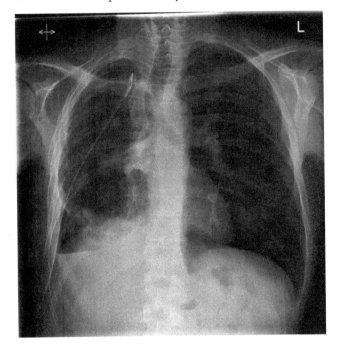

Figure 58.1

Image findings: there is a right-sided intercostal drain, draining the right apical pneumothorax. The white margin of the visceral pleura separated from the parietal pleura can be seen. There is a zone of radio-lucency with absence of vascular markings beyond the visceral pleural margin. Furthermore, a well-defined horizontal fluid level is seen at the base of the right lung. This represents an air-fluid level. This is diagnostic of a hydropneumothrax. Given the clinical history the fluid was likely to be blood – this was confirmed when the chest drain was inserted.

Diagnosis: hydropneumothorax.

Hydropneumothorax is the presence of both air and fluid in the pleural space. The fluid on an erect chest radiograph has a well-defined horizontal superior margin, which usually extends across the whole width of the hemithorax. This occurs at the air/fluid interface.

Causes of hydropneumothorax include:

- trauma – this is the commonest cause of hydropneumothorax. The fluid may be due to blood (haemothorax), chyle (rupture of the thoracic duct) or gastric contents (rupture of the oesophagus)
- spontaneous pneumothorax – commonly, there is a small amount of fluid in the pleural space causing only blunting of the costophrenic angle. Occasionally a moderate haemothorax may develop due to tearing of a pleural adhesion between the visceral and parietal pleura
- bronchopleural fistula – this may result following thoracic surgery, for example, lobectomy
- oesophageal tear/rupture
- iatrogenic – air can be introduced during aspiration of a pleural effusion or following an incorrectly positioned central line
- infection – the presence of gas forming organisms such as tuberculosis and fungi may lead to a hydropneumothorax.

Treatment is by the insertion of a chest drain. When haemothoraces resolve they can leave plaque like areas of pleural calcification which have a similar appearance to asbestos pleural plaques. Unlike asbestos related pleural plaques these are usually unilateral.

Case 59

A 75-year-old gentleman with known carcinoma of the prostate presents with constant generalised back pain, not relieved by analgesia. There is no history of trauma. A bone scan is requested.

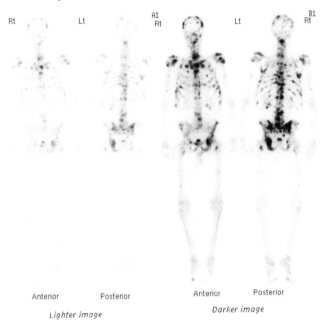

Anterior   Posterior   Anterior   Posterior

Lighter image   *Darker image*

Figure 59.1

Image findings: Figure 59.1 is a whole body bone scan (scintigram) acquired using Tc-99m methylene diphosphonate (MDP), anterior and posterior views. It demonstrates multiple areas of increased uptake of tracer (darker areas) in the ribs, pelvis and spine. The radiologic appearances are due to multiple bony metastases which in this case are from carcinoma of the prostate. Tracer is also seen in the kidneys through which MDP is excreted.

Diagnosis: bone metastases.

Bone scanning is usually performed using Technetium-99m which is a radioactive isotope. This is combined with a diphosphonate compound to create Tc-99m methylene diphosphonate. MDP is injected into the vein of a patient who is then scanned with a gamma camera which detects the radiation emitted. Static or dynamic images may be acquired. Dynamic imaging is performed for suspected osteomyelitis and fractures.

Bone scintigraphy is indicated in the detection of:

- bone metastases
- primary bone tumours
- osteomyelitis
- suspected fractures not clear on plain radiographs (including stress fractures).

Areas of high bone turnover (increased osteoblastic activity) manifests as increased uptake on bone scans (hot spots). Increased bone turnover occurs with metastases, tumours, infection and fractures. However, interpretation of bone scans can be difficult as degenerative arthritis can also appear as hot spots. Bone infarction or lesions which stimulate no osteoblastic response may appear as photopenic areas (cold spots). Notably myeloma may not stimulate osteoblastic activity and can have a normal bone scan.

Bone metastases are common with carcinoma of the prostate and are typically sclerotic, *see* Figure 59.2. But, occasionally they can be lytic. The metastases are predominantly osteoblastic, hence the increased uptake on bone scan. Prostate specific antigen (PSA) is a marker for prostatic cancer and an increase in its level in patients with prostate cancer should raise the suspicion of metastatic spread to the bone.

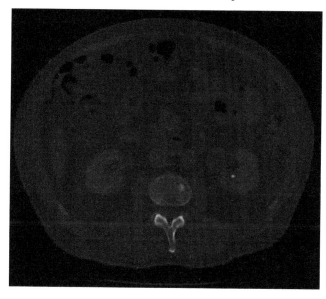

Figure 59.2 Axial CT image on bone windows showing a sclerotic metastasis in a lumbar vertebra due to carcinoma of the prostate.

Case 60

A 45-year-old man with a long history of alcohol abuse presents to his GP with recurrent attacks of epigastric pain radiating to back. He is known to have diabetes mellitus. A plain radiograph of his abdomen is requested.

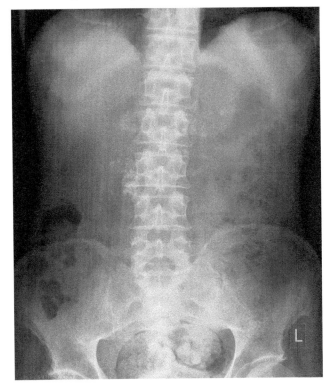

Figure 60.1

Image findings: Figure 60.1 is a plain film of the abdomen revealing multiple speckled areas of high density (foci of white) centrally, at the site corresponding to the pancreas. With the known history of alcohol abuse, these were thought most likely to represent pancreatic calcifications due to chronic pancreatitis.

Diagnosis: chronic pancreatitis.

Chronic pancreatitis is the irreversible inflammatory damage of the pancreas due to recurrent episodes of acute pancreatitis, leading to parenchymal atrophy and fibrosis. Both the exocrine and endocrine functions of the pancreas may be impaired. Clinical diagnosis is often vague, so imaging is employed to confirm the diagnosis.

The commonest causes of acute pancreatitis are alcohol, gallstones, steroids, trauma (including iatrogenic causes, e.g. ERCP). Patients present with an 'acute abdomen' with severe epigastric pain radiating to the back and vomiting. Blood tests show a serum amylase >1000 U/ml.

In chronic pancreatitis, plain film characteristically shows pancreatic calcification, either local or diffuse. CT may show calculi within the ducts or acini of the gland, atrophy of the pancreatic parenchyma, dilation of the main pancreatic duct (usually in a beaded pattern of alternating areas of dilation and constriction) and intra and peripancreatic cysts, *see* Figure 60.2.

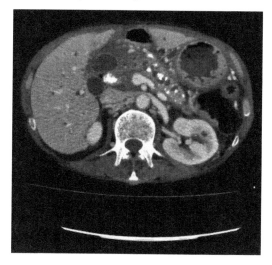

Figure 60.2

Figure 60.2 is an axial contrast enhanced CT of the same patient demonstrating multiple pancreatic calcific foci, which correspond to the calcifications seen on plain film. There are also multiple intra-pancreatic cysts seen as well-defined rounded low attenuation (dark) areas. Atrophy of the gland and dilatation of the pancreatic duct are not evident in this patient.

Figure 60.3 is an axial contrast enhanced image in the same patient during a bout of acute pancreatitis. The pancreas is inflamed and oedematous (hazy grey colour) with a lot of surrounding inflammatory change (surrounding stranding). Ultrasound/CT are useful in identifying the underlying cause of the pancreatitis and also to look for the complications of pancreatitis which can include: pancreatic necrosis, pseudocyst formation, portal vein thrombosis.

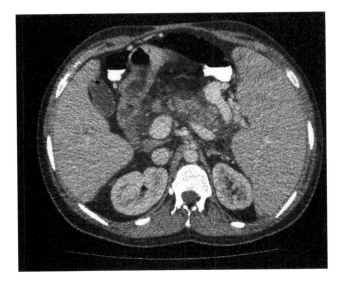

Figure 60.3

Pancreatic calcification is not specific to chronic pancreatitis, but can also occur in hyperparathyroidism, cystic fibrosis, hereditary pancreatitis (calcifications are rounder, larger), pancreatic carcinoma (stellate calcification) and pseudocyst formation (curvilinear calcification).

Case 61

A 70-year-old woman is brought into accident and emergency by an ambulance following a fall at a nursing home. She complains of severe pain in her left hip and is unable to move her left leg.

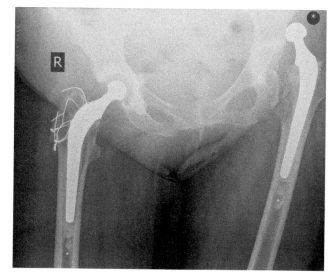

Figure 61.1

Image findings: this an AP radiograph of the pelvis. There are bilateral total hip replacements in-situ. The left hip prosthesis is dislocated posteriorly.

Diagnosis: dislocated left hip.

The hip is a modified ball and socket joint. The femoral head is located deep within the socket of the acetabulum with further stability from a cartilaginous labrum. Hip dislocations in a native hip usually occur secondary to severe trauma as a high force is required to dislocate the joint. There is an increased incidence of posterior hip dislocations following surgical hip replacement, especially in the early period following surgery when even trivial movement such as crossing your legs can cause the femoral head to dislocate posteriorly.

In this example, the patient has had bilateral total hip replacements due to osteoarthritis. Total hip replacements are most commonly performed due to chronic pain and limited mobility from osteoarthritis. They may also be performed following hip fractures, infection or avascular necrosis.

Dislocations of the hip are classified as either anterior, posterior or central depending on the direction of the dislocation. Posterior dislocations account for over 90% of dislocations at the hip. Dislocations are usually easily identified on the AP pelvis view. The position of the dislocation can be determined on an AP view alone.

In a posterior dislocation, *see* Figure 61.1, the femoral head is displaced lateral and superior to the acetabulum. In anterior dislocation of the hip, the femoral head lies medial and inferior to the acetabulum. A central dislocation usually occurs together with a fracture of the acetabulum as the femoral head migrates into the pelvic cavity.

It is essential to assess the neurovascular status of the leg if the hip is dislocated. Common complications from a hip dislocation include sciatic nerve injury, vascular injury, arthritis and avascular necrosis.

Case 62

A 30-year-old cyclist attends accident and emergency having been knocked down by a car. He has a swollen and painful left knee. Plain radiographs of the knee are requested.

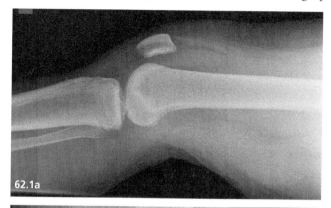

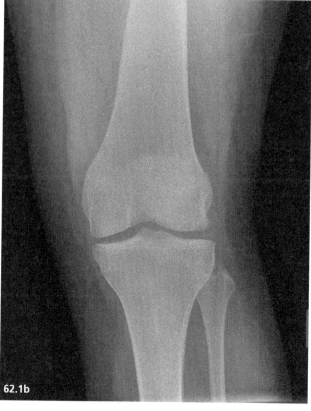

Figure 62.1a, b

Image findings: AP and cross-table lateral views of the left knee are shown in Figures 62.1a and b. The lateral radiograph shows the presence a lipohaemarthrosis demonstrated by a fat-fluid level in the suprapatellar bursa. A definite fracture site is not visible.

Diagnosis: lipohaemarthrosis.

The presence of a lipohaemarthrosis (fat-fluid level) on a cross-table lateral view of the knee indicates the presence of a significant intra-articular fracture, such as a tibial plateau fracture. The patient should be managed as having an intra-articular fracture of the knee even if an obvious fracture site is not found.

In an effusion of the knee joint, the suprapatellar bursa fills with fluid. This is shown in Figure 62.2 by the presence of an oval density that displaces the suprapatellar fat pad anterior to the distal femur.

In lipohaemarthrosis (*see* Figure 62.1a), fat is released from the bone marrow as a result of the intra-articular fracture. This fat layers on top of the underlying fluid (blood) resulting in the fat-fluid level. This can be better appreciated on MRI which can more clearly differentiate between the two.

There are a number of processes that can lead to the development of a knee effusion, these include:

- fractures around the knee joint
- soft tissue injury including injuries to the menisci and cruciate ligaments
- patella subluxation/dislocation
- septic arthritis of the knee
- rheumatic conditions such as rheumatoid arthritis, gout and pseudogout
- neoplasms.

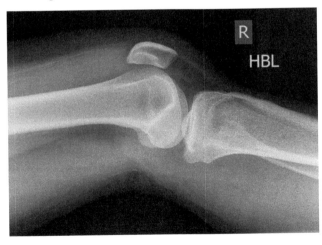

Figure 62.2 Lateral knee radiograph showing a large effusion.

Case 63

A 25-year-old lady who developed a traumatic ulcer at the dorsum of her right middle finger complains of worsening pain, redness and swelling of her finger two weeks after the injury. Radiographs of her finger are obtained.

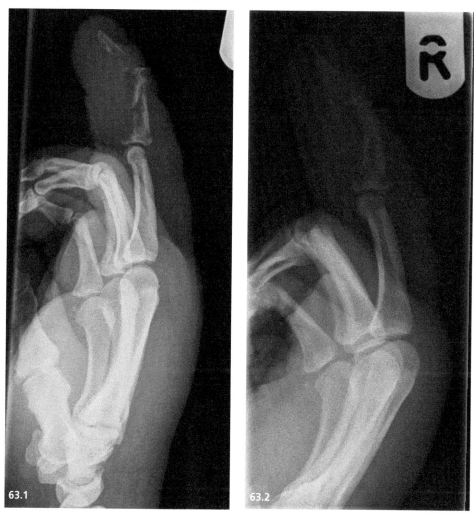

Figures 63.1 and 63.2

Image findings: there is diffuse marked soft tissue swelling of the finger. Multiple lytic lesions of the terminal and middle phalanges of the finger can be seen. There is destruction of the cortex of the phalanges and there is gas in the soft tissues (seen as a focus of black). This is a case of osteomyelitis of the finger.

Diagnosis: osteomyelitis.

Infectious organisms can reach the bone via three mechanisms:

1   haematogenous spread
2   a contiguous source, e.g. from the soft tissues
3   direct implantation, e.g. trauma or surgery.

In children, the commonest site for osteomyelitis to develop is the metaphysis. In adults, infection can develop in any part of a bone. There is no reliable way to radiographically exclude a focus of osteomyelitis. If a bony sequestrum is present, osteomyelitis should be strongly considered.
   Radiographic signs of osteomyelitis:

- soft tissue oedema (occurs within 24–48 hours)
- destructive lytic lesion (7–10 days)
- destruction of cortical and medullary bone and the formation of periosteal new bone in an effort to wall off infection (2–6 weeks)
- sequestrum (latin: to seclude) which is a focus of dead avascular bone (6–8 weeks)
- the sequestrum can be surrounded by an involucrum (latin: to wrap or cover). This represents a sheath of periosteal new bone
- draining sinus tract (chronic osteomyelitis).

The radiographic pattern of osteomyelitis may resemble Langerhans cell histiocytosis and Ewing sarcoma. Because the earliest positive radiographic changes of osteomyelitis may not be evident for at least 10 days after the start of infection, a bone scan or MRI may be performed for earlier detection. Prompt diagnosis and treatment of osteomyelitis is essential for an optimal response to antibiotics.

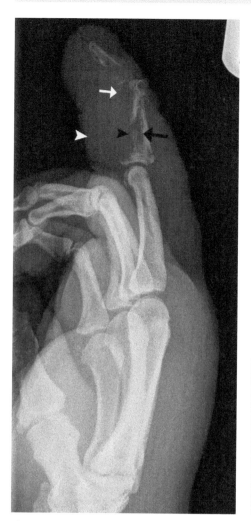
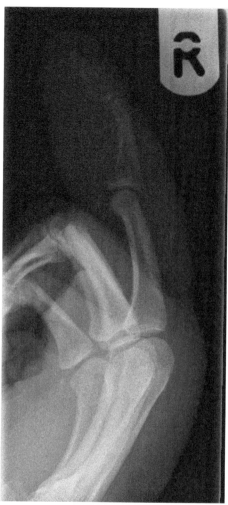

Figure 63.3 Radiograph of the right index finger two weeks after the injury. There are lytic lesions (black arrow), destruction of the cortex (black arrowhead), gas (white arrow) and soft tissue swelling (white arrowhead) consistent with osteomyelitis.

Figure 63.4 Radiograph of the right index finger three weeks after the injury.

Case 64

A 48-year-old female presented to rapid access chest pain clinic with a three-month history of atypical chest pain. The pain was not particularly related to exercise. There was no associated shortness of breath. She smoked 10 cigarettes per day for the last 20 years. She had no history of hypertension or diabetes and had no family history of cardiovascular disease. The patient was referred for an exercise test but unfortunately could not manage this due to a longstanding ankle injury. She was therefore referred for a cardiac CT angiogram.

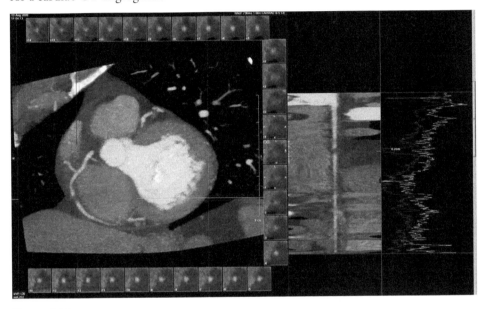

Figure 64.1

Image findings: the reformatted sagittal cardiac CT image shows a tight stenosis in the mid right coronary artery (RCA).

Diagnosis: RCA stenosis.

Exercise tolerance testing has been previously used as the first line investigation to determine whether or not chest pain is due to coronary artery disease. Patients are required to exercise on a treadmill following a set (e.g. Bruce) protocol. There is increase in the exercise work over a 12 minute period and the patient is monitored for ECG changes and for symptoms. The problem with this test is that it is has a relatively poor sensitivity and there are groups of patients who are unable to exercise. Therefore other methods of investigation for ischaemic heart disease involve using a drug, e.g. dobutamine or adenosine to increase the work of the heart without the patient needing to physically exercise. These include:

- nuclear medicine stress testing – MIBI scan
- stress echo
- stress cardiac MRI.

Another alternative is cardiac CT angiography – this is a relatively new technology which offers a coronary artery angiogram with a contrast injection in the arm. It has the advantage of being a quick test and is less invasive than a conventional angiogram.

After the cardiac CT the patient was referred for an urgent interventional procedure and had a conventional angiogram with an angioplasty and stent procedure.

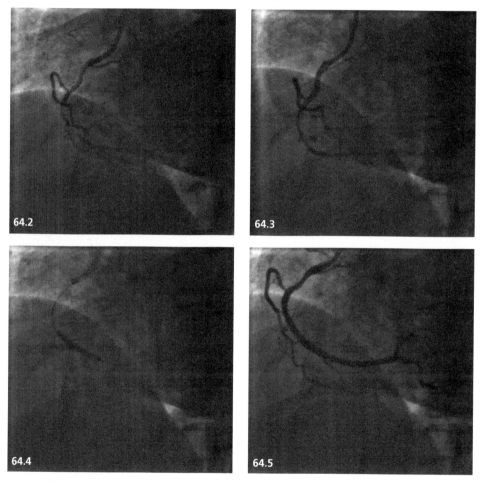

Figures 64.2, 64.3, 64.4, 64.5 Images acquired from the same patient following a diagnostic coronary angiogram, followed by angioplasty of the right coronary artery.

Case 65

A 55-year-old woman is brought into the emergency department with a headache and dysphasia. She has previously had a mastectomy for breast cancer. A pre and post contrast CT head scan is requested.

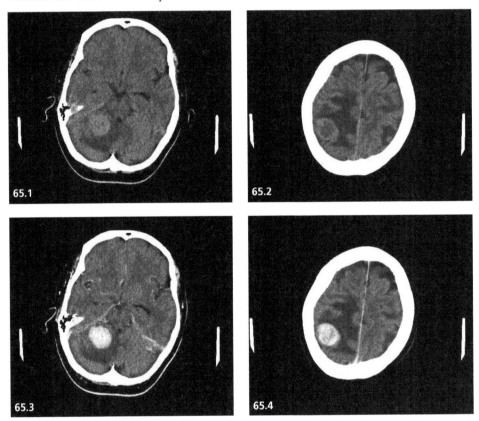

Figures 65.1, 65.2, 65.3 and 65.4

Image findings: the non-contrasted axial CT head images (Figures 65.1 and 65.2) demonstrate well-defined rounded lesions of mixed attenuation of varying sizes in the right cerebellum and the right parietal lobe. There is vasogenic oedema (dark areas) surrounding these lesions. These lesions enhance avidly on the CT scan following the administration of contrast (Figures 65.3 and 65.4).

Diagnosis: cerebral metastases.

Cerebral metastases are the most common intracranial tumour accounting for 40% of all intracranial neoplasms in adults. The majority of cerebral metastases are multifocal with approximately 30% solitary at presentation. Below is a list of the common primary malignancies that metastasise to the brain:

- bronchial carcinoma
- breast carcinoma
- colon carcinoma
- renal cell carcinoma
- melanoma
- choriocarcinoma.

Cerebral metastases on MRI and CT imaging are commonly seen as multiple lesions located at the gray-white matter interface. Metastases usually appear as hypodense lesions (dark) on non-contrasted CT scans that enhance uniformly with contrast, as shown in this case. They tend to vary in size with surrounding vasogenic oedema. Exceptions to this are haemorrhagic metastases which will appear hyperdense on a non-contrasted scan and enhance avidly following contrast. Haemorrhagic cerebral metastases are typically encountered in melanoma, thyroid carcinoma and renal cell carcinoma.

When rounded rim enhancing lesions are identified in the brain, it can be sometimes difficult to distinguish metastases from brain abscesses. History, examination and bloods can help – look for signs of pyrexia, raised WCC, raised CRP, signs of sepsis, rapid symptom onset (abscess) or weight loss. In immunocompromised patients, toxoplasmosis and lymphoma can also give similar CT appearances.

Case 66

A 60-year-old woman presents to the emergency department with slurred speech and right sided upper and lower limb weakness.

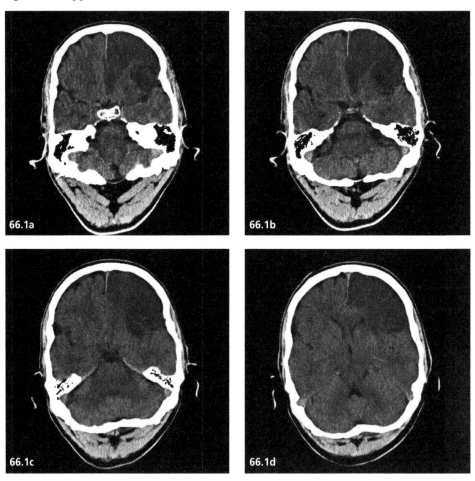

Figures 66.1a, b, c, d

Image findings: there is a wedge shaped area of low attenuation in the left frontal lobe extending to the cortical surface involving the white and grey matter. No midline shift. Features are consistent with a left anterior cerebral artery infarct.

Diagnosis: left anterior cerebral artery territory infarction.

A cerebrovascular accident (CVA) or a stroke as it is commonly known describes the sudden onset of an acute neurological deficit. A stroke results from a sudden interruption of the blood supply to part of the brain. The presenting signs and symptoms of a stroke vary in severity depending on the location and size of the stroke. Symptoms of a stroke include limb weakness, numbness, blurred vision, slurred speech, confusion and fitting. Some 80% of strokes are ischaemic in nature and 20% haemorrhagic. Cerebral ischaemia signifies a reduction in the blood supply to the brain whereas cerebral infarction refers to permanent brain damage as a consequence of ischaemia. The term transient ischaemic attack (TIA) is used to define an acute neurological disturbance that completely resolves within 24 hours. The common causes of a stroke are listed below:

- cerebral infarction (80%)
  - ∘ thromboembolic disease secondary to atherosclerosis (60%)
  - ∘ cardiogenic emboli (15%)
  - ∘ other (5%)
- primary intracranial haemorrhage (15%)
- vasospasm secondary to non-traumatic subarachnoid haemorrhage (4%)
- venous occlusion (1%).

A CT scan should be performed within 24 hours if a stroke is suspected. An immediate CT head scan is warranted if thrombolysis is being considered, or the GCS is less than 13 or if the patient is taking anti-coagulants. A CT scan is the initial modality of choice as the treatment and management of an ischaemic stroke differs from that of a haemorrhagic stroke. Thrombolysis should be considered in an acute ischaemic stroke if the patient presents within three hours from the onset of symptoms and an intracranial haemorrhage has been excluded. A neurosurgical opinion should be requested in the presence of a haemorrhagic stroke.

CT is more sensitive than MRI in detecting acute blood/haemorrhage. However MRI is superior to CT in the early detection of cerebral ischaemia, particularly diffusion weighted imaging. CT scan is frequently normal in early stroke. Common signs seen on a CT head scan include loss of the grey-white matter interface, areas of low attenuation extending to the cortex and a hyperdense clot in the middle cerebral artery (MCA) commonly known as the hyperdense MCA sign.

Case 67

A 40-year-old man with an 18 month history of back pain is seen by his GP. The back pain radiates down the patient's left leg with numbness affecting his left foot. Plain radiographs and a MRI of the lumbosacral spine are requested.

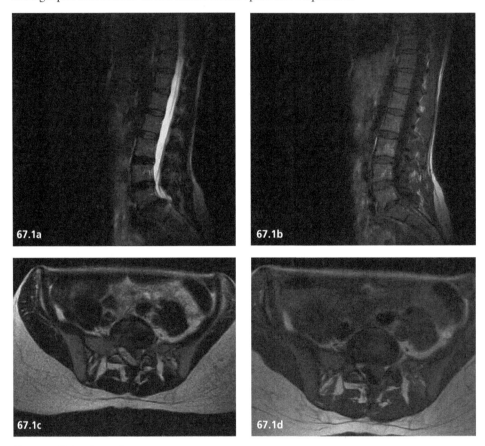

Figures 67.1a, b, c, d

Image findings: there is dehydration of the lower lumbar L3/4, L4/5 and L5/S1 discs shown as decreased signal intensity (dark) on the T2 weighted images (Figures 67.1a and c). The intervertebral disc space normally increases in size down the lumbar spine, however, on this MRI there is narrowing of the intervertebral disc space at the levels of L4/L5 and L5/S1. At the level of L5/S1 there is a focal left paracentral disc herniation compressing the nerve roots.

Diagnosis: degenerative disc disease with a focal left paracentral disc herniation at L5/S1 level.

Approximately 80% of individuals will experience lower back pain (LBP) during their lifetime. The majority of cases are acute, benign and self-limiting requiring no imaging. Diagnostic imaging of the lumbar spine is only performed if surgery is being considered or if the patient has additional worrying presenting signs or symptoms such as:

- red flag symptoms – unable to pass urine, decreased anal tone which suggest a cauda equine syndrome
- neurological deficit
- >50 years of age
- trauma
- history of malignancy
- fever.

Degenerative disc disease is the most common cause for LBP. Other causes include spondylolysis +/- spondylolisthesis, malignancy, infection such as osteomyelitis/TB or an epidural abscess.

It is usual practice to request a plain radiograph of the lumbar spine in the first instance to exclude a traumatic fracture to the spine or detect structural abnormalities such as a pars defect (fracture of the pars intraarticularis which gives the collar to the Scottie dog on the lateral thoracic spine images), spondylolisthesis (anterior slip of one vertebral body on the one below – this is most commonly seen at L5/S1 level) or bony degenerative changes. MRI imaging of the spine is the optimal modality to assess for the presence of intervertebral disc disease, spinal canal stenosis and spinal cord abnormalities, infection and neoplasm.

Disc herniation on MRI can broadly be classified as:

- generalised disc bulge – increase in diameter of the whole disc
- disc protrusion – a focal disc bulge with a wide base
- disc prolapse – A focal disc base with a narrow base/separated disc fragment.

Signs of degenerative disc disease on a plain film include loss of intervertebral disc height, marginal osteophytes and sclerotic vertebral end plates, *see* Figures 67.2a and b.

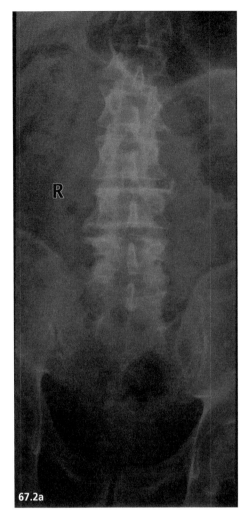

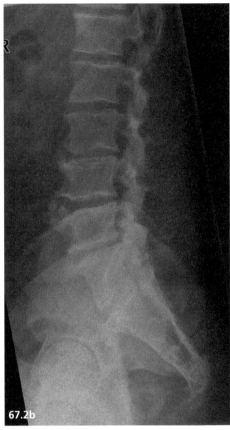

Figures 67.2 a, b Anteroposterior and lateral image of the lumbar spine show facet joint degenerative disease, loss of intervertebral disc height, end plate sclerosis and multiple osteophytes.

Case 68

A child attends the emergency department following a fall. He complains of pain, swelling and tenderness of his right forearm.

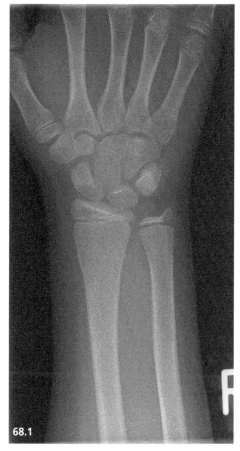

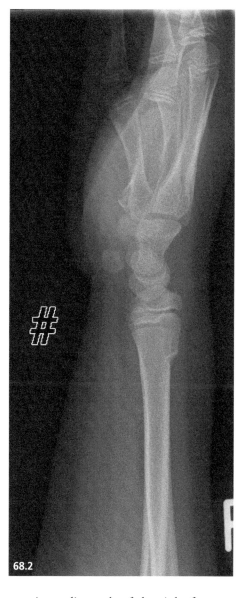

Figures 68.1 and 68.2

Image findings: Figure 68.1 is an anteroposterior radiograph of the right forearm revealing a subtle cortical bulge of the right distal radius (there is a slight bump in the cortex). The lateral view (Figure 68.2) shows buckling of the cortex and angular deformity of the distal radius more clearly. This is diagnostic of a buckle fracture, also known as a 'torus' fracture.

Diagnosis: buckle fracture.

Children's bones are more elastic than adult bones and the periosteum is thicker. Therefore children's bones tend to bow or bend before breaking. Buckle fractures of the radius and ulna occur commonly following a fall on an outstretched hand. Radiographs show bulging or a slight bump of the cortex, which can often be subtle.

Other types of fracture which can occur in children are:

- **greenstick fracture** – usually results from an angulation force. There is a break in the cortex on one side of the bone. The opposite cortex appears intact (histologically in fact, there is a fracture of the other cortex that may be invisible or impacted)
- **plastic bowing fracture** – the bone bends/bows with no obvious break in the cortex-microfractures develop but there is no visible fracture line.

Case 69

A 75-year-old man who is a known hypertensive attends the emergency department with sudden onset of severe tearing chest pain, radiating to the back. On examination his peripheral pulses and blood pressures are unequal. A chest X-ray is obtained.

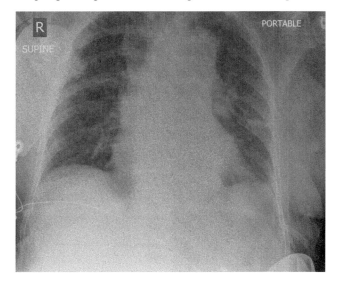

Figure 69.1

Image findings: Figure 69.1 is a chest X-ray demonstrating a widened mediastinum, despite being an AP film. The mediastinum is widened to greater than 8 cm. The clinical findings together with radiographic appearances suggest an aortic dissection and an urgent CT is obtained.

Diagnosis: aortic dissection.

WIDENING OF THE MEDIASTINUM

The mediastinum is the space between the two lungs bounded by the mediastinal pleura. It extends from the sternum to the vertebral column and from the thoracic inlet to the diaphragm. It contains the heart, the great vessels of the heart, oesophagus, trachea, lymph nodes and thymus. A widened mediastinum is one with a width greater than 8 cm on posteroanterior chest X-ray. Be wary that the mediastinum may appear falsely widened if the radiograph is taken in the anteroposterior supine position.

Differential causes of mediastinal widening include: Aortic aneurysm, aortic rupture, thoracic vertebrae fracture, lymphadenopathy, mediastinal mass, e.g. thymoma, teratoma, pericardial effusion, oesophageal rupture.

AORTIC DISSECTION

Aortic dissection occurs when blood splits the media of the aortic wall. The aortic intima and adventitia become separated by blood. Aortic dissection consequently leads to occlusion of branches of the aorta. It occurs by two mechanisms:

1 via a tear in the intima – this is the most common cause. Predisposing factors include cystic medial degeneration and hypertension
2 primary haemorrhage into the aortic wall – bleeding of the vasa vasorum causing intramural haematoma.

Other predisposing risk factors include Marfan syndrome, Ehlers-Danlos and pregnancy.

The chest X-ray is not sensitive or specific for the diagnosis of aortic dissection. Abnormal findings include widening of the mediastinum, left pleural effusion, atelectasis of the left lower lobe, irregular contour to the aorta and displaced calcification. CT is highly sensitive and specific. Findings on CT include opacification of two channels (attributed to a true and a false lumen), displaced intimal calcification, intimal flap and an entry tear, *see* Figures 69.2a and b.

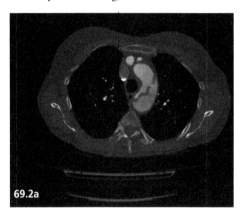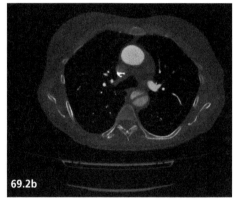

Figure 69.2a, b Axial contrast enhanced CT of the thorax revealing an intimal flap extending along the aortic arch and descending aorta, creating two channels (a true and false lumen). There is opacification of both channels with contrast although the channel nearer to the spine is probably the false channel as it has a lower attenuation value (less bright), reflecting slower flow.

There are two classification systems for aortic dissection – the DeBakey and Stanford. The Stanford classification system helps decide treatment. Type A dissections require surgery, while type B dissections may be managed medically.

1 **Type A (60%)** – ascending aorta and arch. This type of dissection is treated by emergency surgery as these can be complicated by rupture into the pericardium leading to caradic tamponade.
2 **Type B (40%)** – descending aorta only (begins beyond the left subclavian artery).

Case 70

Two different patients attend the emergency department both following falls. They complain of severe left hip pain and reduced movement of the hip.

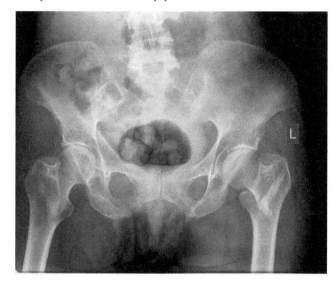

Figure 70.1

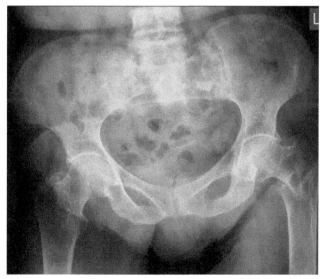

Figure 70.2

Image findings: Figure 70.1 is an anteroposterior pelvic X-ray demonstrating a displaced fracture of the neck of the left femur. Compared to the right hip, the cortex of the neck of the left femur is not smooth and there is a step. There is also an area of sclerosis (white) at the fracture site due to impacted bone. This is an intracapsular fracture involving the femoral neck.

Figure 70.2 is a pelvic X-ray in the second patient demonstrating an intertrochanteric fracture of the left femur. There is a visible fracture line (black) extending between the greater and lesser trochanters. The cortex of the proximal femur is discontinuous and there is a large step at the intertrochanteric region.

Diagnosis: fractures of the proximal femur.

Most fractures of the proximal femur occur in the elderly whose bones are osteoporotic and can occur following a minor injury or fall. On examination the leg may be shortened and externally rotated. Fractures of the proximal femur can be classified as intracapsular and extracapsular depending on the level.

Intracapsular fractures involve the femoral head and neck:

- capital
- subcapital
- transcervical
- basicervical.

Extracapsular fractures involve the trochanters:

- intertrochanteric (extending from the greater trochanter to the lesser trochanter)
- subtrochanteric.

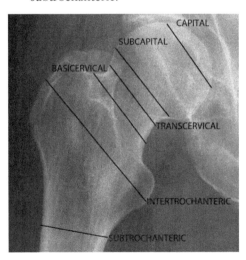

Figures 70.3 Diagram to show classification of levels of fractures of the proximal femur.

The risk of avascular necrosis is more common following an intracapsular fracture. This is because the majority of the blood supply to the femoral head is from the circumflex femoral arteries which form a ring about the neck of the femur. Branches ascend along the femoral neck to the femoral head. Intracapsular fractures tend to interrupt this blood supply. Fractures more distally involving the trochanteric region are at less risk of avascular necrosis because there is an alternate blood supply from muscles around the trochanters. There are many classification systems for femoral neck fractures. The Garden system is commonly used and is based upon the degree of displacement of the femoral head.

Case 71

A 65-year-old woman with a history of recurrent falls is admitted to accident and emergency with a fluctuating conscious level, headache and vomiting. She has a GCS of 11. An urgent CT head is requested.

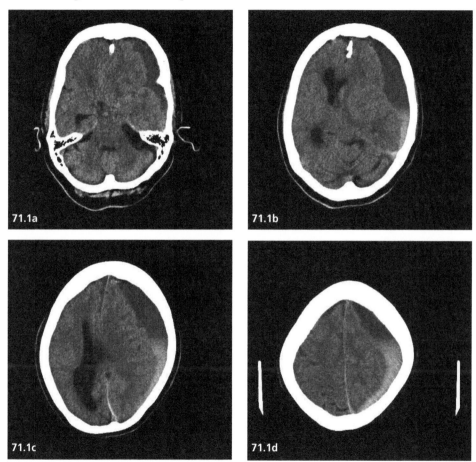

Figures 71.1a, b, c, d

Image findings: the selected images from an axial CT head scan show the presence of an acute on chronic subdural haematoma overlying the left cerebral convexity. There is an extra-axial fluid collection with layering of chronic blood (low attenuation/dark) over the acute blood (high attenuation/bright). Subdural haematomas are typically crescent shaped extra-axial collections. If this was an acute subdural haematoma, the collection in the subdural space would be only of high attenuation (bright). In this case, there is also a mass effect resulting in compression of the ipsilateral ventricle and midline shift. There are also signs of hydrocephalus demonstrated by dilatation of the temporal horn of the right lateral ventricle.

Diagnosis: acute on chronic left sided subdural haematoma.

This case demonstrates the typical findings of an acute subdural haematoma on CT. A subdural haematoma represents venous bleeding from torn cortical veins in the subdural space which lies between the dura and arachnoid mater. Subdural haematomas are commonly caused by acceleration/deceleration injuries from falling over and road traffic collisions. They are also commonly seen in patients suffering from recurrent falls, alcoholics, epileptics, those with abnormal coagulation and patients taking aspirin or warfarin.

The National Institute for Clinical Excellence (NICE) has produced guidelines for the management of patients presenting with a head injury and the circumstances in which an urgent CT head scan should be requested. An immediate CT scan will facilitate the early detection of treatable intracranial bleeding requiring surgical intervention thus preventing long term neurological damage. A CT scan rather than a MRI should be requested as acute haemorrhage is not readily detectable on MRI. Due to the number of patients that present with a head injury and the fact that a CT scan involves ionising radiation, it would not be feasible to scan every patient unless there is a high index of suspicion. The NICE guidelines are summarised below.

Indications for an urgent CT head scan:

- GCS<13 when first assessed in emergency department
- GCS<15 when assessed in emergency department two hours after injury
- suspected open or depressed skull fracture
- sign of fracture at skull base (haemotympanum, 'panda' eyes, CSF leakage from ears or nose, Battle's sign)
- post-traumatic seizure
- focal neurological deficit
- >1 episode of vomiting
- amnesia of events >30 minutes before impact.

Patients who are diagnosed with subdural bleeds need to be urgently discussed with the neurosurgical team. Urgent surgical intervention is required, particularly when there are signs of hydrocephalus. Surgical treatment with burr holes or craniotomy to relieve pressure and to evacuate clot can lead to a full recovery.

Case 72

A 25-year-old man is brought into the emergency department by ambulance following an assault with a baseball bat. His GCS had been 15/15 since the assault but rapidly deteriorated to 9/15 with nausea and vomiting soon after arrival to the emergency department.

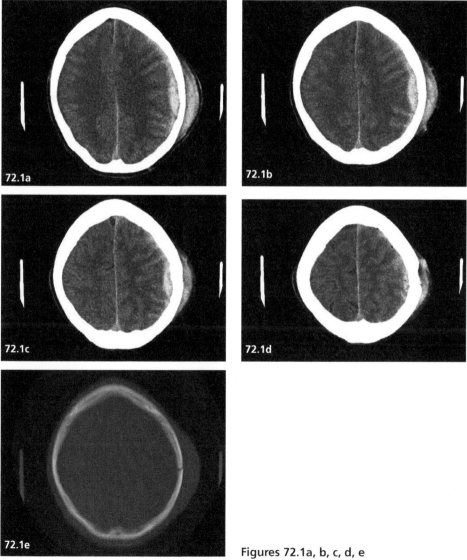

Figures 72.1a, b, c, d, e

Image findings: these images are from an axial CT head scan. There is a left-sided extradural haematoma demonstrated by a well-defined biconvex extra-axial collection of high attenuation (bright). Figure 72.1e shows the cranial vault windowed to bone settings. A lucent fracture line through the temporal bone overlying the extradural haematoma is evident with marked swelling of the overlying scalp. On the very superior CT brain images (*see* Figure 72.1d) it is possible to see locules of gas within the skull cavity which is a consequence of the fracture. A large surrounding subcutaneous haematoma is also demonstrated.

Diagnosis: left-sided extradural haematoma.

A lucid interval following a head injury is a hallmark feature of an extradural haematoma. An extradural haematoma represents blood in the space between the inner table of the cranial vault and the dura. The majority of extradural haematomas are arterial in origin caused by disruption of the middle meningeal artery and occur in the temporal or temporoparietal region. The developing haematoma strips the dura from the inner table of the vault forming a lentiform shaped collection that does not cross cranial suture lines. Over 85% of patients will have an associated fracture as demonstrated in this case. Venous extradural haematomas are uncommon and tend to occur as a result of disrupted dural venous sinuses.

It is essential to assess for features of raised intracranial pressure and mass effect which appear as midline shift, effacement of the sulci and ventricular dilatation. Between 30% and 50% of patients will have other injuries visible on the CT scan such as a contrecoup subdural haematoma and cerebral contusions. A contrecoup injury represents a brain injury directly opposite the site of impact.

In the presence of any intracranial haemorrhage, an urgent neurosurgical opinion should be requested as an emergency craniotomy and evacuation of the clot can improve morbidity and mortality. *See* Case 71 for the recommended NICE guidelines of the acute management of a head injury.

Case 73

A 70-year-old man has an abdominal radiograph taken following a procedure performed in the interventional radiology suite. He was originally admitted with a recent diagnosis of a bladder tumour and deranged renal function.

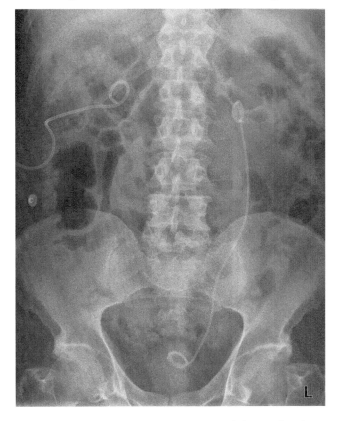

Figure 73.1

Image findings: this is an AP supine abdominal radiograph. There is a left ureteric JJ-stent and a right nephrostomy in-situ. The left ureteric stent appears to be correctly sited with the distal end in the bladder.

Diagnosis: right-sided nephrostomy and left ureteric stent.

Nephrostomy is the term used to describe the presence of a tube, stent or catheter communicating between the skin surface and the renal pelvis or calyx. The insertion of a nephrostomy is usually performed by an interventional radiologist under fluoroscopic or ultrasound guidance.

A nephrostomy tube is usually inserted to facilitate the drainage of urine and to relieve a hydronephrosis caused by an obstructed renal tract. Hydronephrosis is defined as a dilatation of the renal pelvis and calyces usually caused by an obstruction to the flow of urine occurring either in the ureter, bladder or the bladder outflow tract. An obstructed system can then become infected and result in systemic infection – therefore this needs to be relieved urgently. Ultrasound is the initial imaging modality of choice to investigate urinary symptoms and abnormal renal function. Figure 73.2 shows the typical appearances of a hydronephrosis on ultrasound. The anechoic (black) areas of the kidney represents a dilated renal pelvis and calyces. The site of obstruction can be determined by the presence of either unilateral or bilateral hydronephrosis. If the hydronephrosis is unilateral, it is likely that the obstruction occurs within the ureter of the same side. (Figure 73.3 is a coronal CT reformatted image showing a large 2 cm stone obstructing the left ureter.) If there is bilateral hydronephrosis, the obstruction is most likely in the bladder or outflow tract.

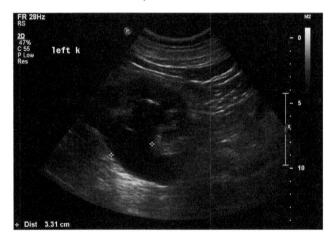

Figure 73.2

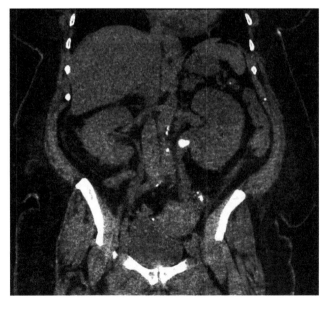

Figure 73.3

A nephrostomy is also performed to gain access to the upper urinary tracts for a number of surgical procedures such as percutaneous nephrolithotomy/PCNL (renal stone removal) and anterograde JJ stent insertion.

Ureteric stents, such as in Figure 73.1, are usually inserted to manage ureteric obstruction caused by ureteric calculi, ureteric strictures or extrinsic compression. Retrograde ureteric stent insertion is performed by urologists inserting the stent through the ureteric orifice during a bladder cystoscopy. Anterograde ureteric stent insertion is performed by an interventional radiologist. The procedure involves puncturing a middle/lower pole calyx percutaneously and manipulating a guidewire through the renal pelvis and ureter into the bladder. A JJ-stent is then passed across the guidewire and deployed into the ureter. It is usual practice to leave a covering nephrostomy at the puncture site which is removed a few days later. The procedure is usually performed under sedation and local anaesthesia. The main complications of the procedure are sepsis, damage to the renal tracts and vascular injury.

Case 74

A 50-year-old lady is referred for an ultrasound scan of her kidneys due to deteriorating renal function. She has no prior history of kidney disease. She denies haematuria.

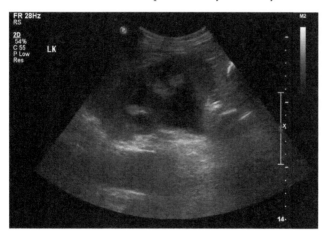

Figure 74.1

Image findings: longitudinal renal ultrasound shows a dilated calyx communicating with a dilated renal pelvis consistent with hydronephrosis.

Diagnosis: hydronephrosis.

The kidney is divided into the outer cortex and an inner medulla. The medulla is further divided into a number of renal pyramids, which are conical in shape. The apex of each pyramid forms a papilla. The renal pelvis is the expanded upper end of the ureter. Extensions of the pelvis, termed the calyces, extend towards the papilla of each pyramid and collect the urine.

Hydronephrosis is defined as dilatation of the upper urinary tract. Ultrasound is a good method of investigation for screening of hydronephrosis. Ultrasound shows a dilated renal pelvis communicating with anechoic (black) fluid-filled calyces, *see* Figure 74.2. There may be renal enlargement. Hydronephrosis can be graded as mild, moderate and severe. It is worth noting that an extrarenal pelvis can be mistaken for a hydronephrotic kidney. This is where the renal pelvis lies predominantly outside of the renal sinus. A parapelvic cyst can also be mistaken for hydronephrosis.

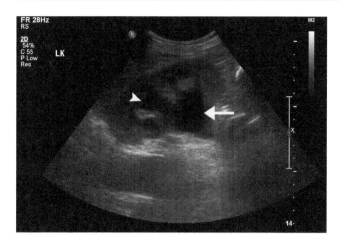

Figure 74.2 Ultrasound image of the left kidney shows a dilated renal pelvis (arrow) and upper pole calyx (arrowhead).

Causes of hydronephrosis to consider include:

- obstruction. This can be due to a stone, stricture, tumour or extrinsic compression. Extrinsic compression can occur for example due to a pelvic mass. Figures 74.3 and 74.4 shows reformatted CT images of bilateral hydronephrosis more marked on the left and massive distension of the bladder. This was as a consequence of prostatic hypertrophy and subsequent outflow obstruction
- reflux nephropathy
- distended bladder
- pregnancy
- diabetes insipidus.

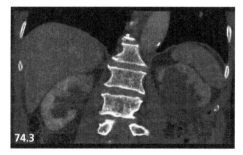

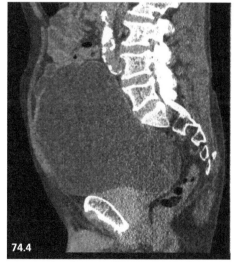

Figures 74.3 and 74.4 Reformatted CT images show bilateral hydronephrosis and bladder distension due to obstruction from prostatic hypertrophy.

Case 75

A 20-year-old girl presented to accident and emergency following a fall on the icy pavement. She landed on her left hand and is now complaining of pain at the medial aspect of her left wrist. On examination she is very tender in the 'anatomical snuff box'. The following series of films was requested by the casualty officer.

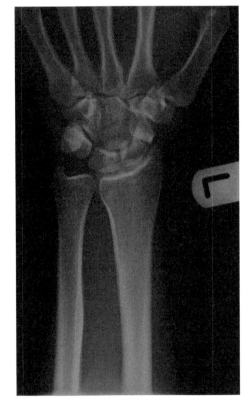

Figure 75.1

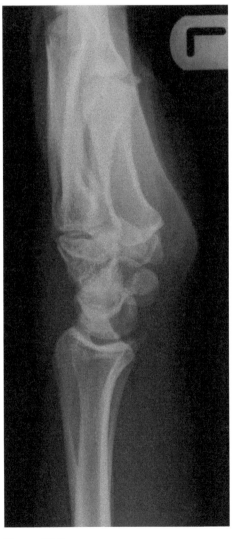

Figure 75.2

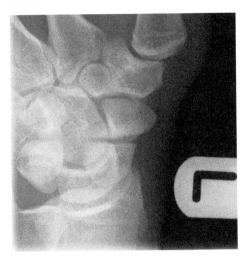

Figure 75.3

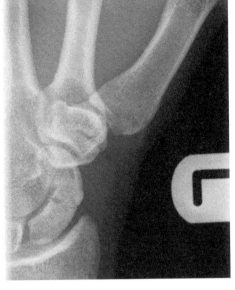

Figure 75.4

Image findings: the 'scaphoid views' series of radiographs show a fracture through the waist of the scaphoid bone.

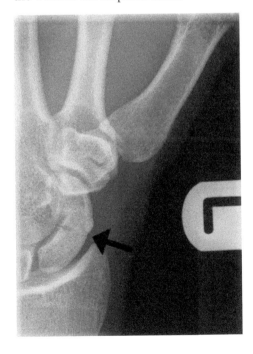

Figure 75.5 Scaphoid fracture (arrow).

Diagnosis: scaphoid fracture.

Scaphoid fractures typically present with anatomical snuff box tenderness. They are the most common of the carpal bone fractures and typically occur due to a fall on an out-stretched hand in the young adult population.

As the blood supply to the proximal pole of the scaphoid enters at the scaphoid waist, the proximal pole is at risk for avascular necrosis if the bloody supply is interrupted at the waist or proximal pole by a fracture. It is therefore essential that all of these fractures are identified and treated. Unfortunately they can be difficult to detect on the initial radiograph. In order to optimise their detection it is necessary to perform a full scaphoid series of radiographs (as shown in this case). If the initial X-rays are normal it is also essential that the patient be followed up. Commonly patients are put in a plaster cast and reviewed with repeat radiographs in 7–10 days. By day 5–10 post injury often the fracture line will be more evident due to bone resorption.

If there is a high clinical suspicion of a scaphoid fracture but even repeat radiographs are normal then other imaging modalities can be used to confirm or exclude the diagnosis. These would include:

- bone scan – a fracture would take up isotope and would appear as a black spot of increased uptake
- CT – the fracture line could be visualised
- MRI.

Case 76

A nine-year-old boy is brought to accident and emergency following a fall from a trampoline. He is complaining of severe pain in his left elbow which is very bruised and swollen on examination. He is unable to move it. The following X-rays were obtained.

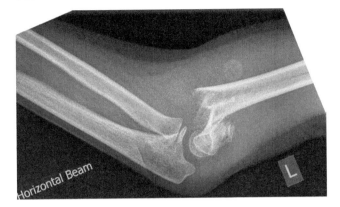

Figure 76.1

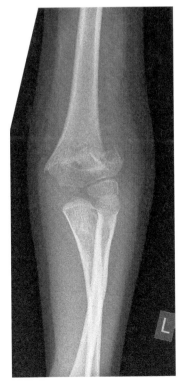

Figure 76.2

Image findings: the frontal and lateral radiographs of the left elbow show a markedly displaced supracondylar fracture of the left distal humerus. There is also marked associated soft tissue swelling around the left elbow.

Diagnosis: supracondylar fracture.

Supracondylar fractures are the most common elbow fractures in children, and they can be subtle and easily missed (although not in this case where the bony fragments are markedly displaced). It is important to follow the cortex of each bone to ensure there are no breaks or steps in order to exclude a fracture. Figure 76.3 and 76.4 demonstrate a much more subtle supracondylar fracture. The fracture line is barely visible on the anteroposterior view (*see* Figure 76.4) but is more easily seen on the lateral view (*see* Figure 76.3).

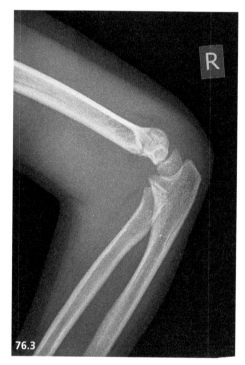

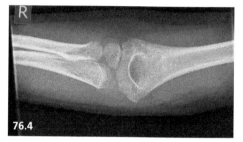

Figures 76.3 and 76.4 Lateral and AP elbow images show a subtle supracondylar fracture.

When looking at an elbow film it is important to assess the *anterior humeral line*. This is a line which runs along the anterior surface of the humerus on the lateral view. In a normal elbow almost one third of the capitellum (distal humeral growth plate) lies anterior to this line, while this is not the case with a supracondylar fracture. Figure 76.5 shows a normal elbow.

A complicating factor in the assessment of paediatric radiographs is the presence of the growth plates/ossification centres. Six separate ossification centres appear at the elbow between birth and 12 years of age. The order of their appearance can be remembered by the acronym CRITOL (**C**apitellum, **R**adial head, **I**nternal (medial) epicondyle, **T**rochlear, **O**lecranon and **L**ateral (external) epicondyle). Avulsion fractures of the internal epicondyle ossification centre are another common injury in the paediatric population and it is important to recognise that if the trochlear ossification centre is present, then the internal epicondyle should also be visualised in its normal position.

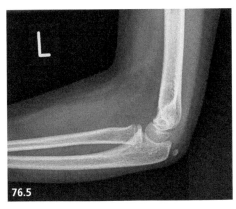

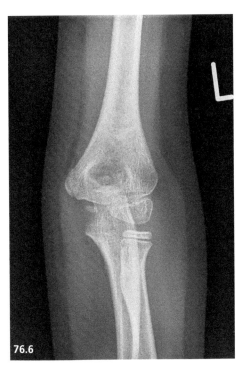

Figures 76.5 and 76.6 Lateral and AP images of a normal elbow showing capitellum, radial head, internal (medial) epicondyle and trochlear and olecranon. The lateral epicondyle has not developed yet.

Case 77

A 16-year-old male presented to accident and emergency following a fall whilst playing football. He had landed on his outstretched left arm and was complaining of pain in the mid left forearm. On examination there was swelling and bruising of the forearm with tenderness along the ulna in particular. The following X-rays were obtained.

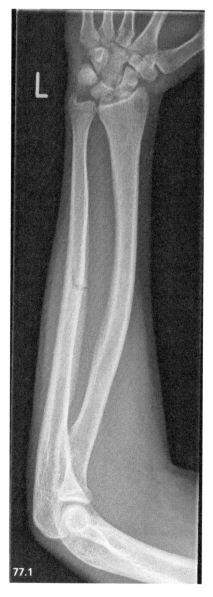

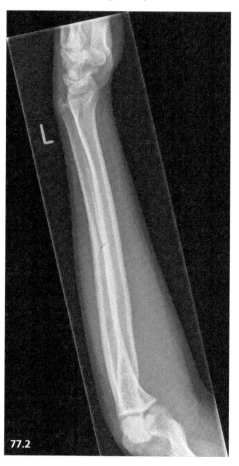

Figures 77.1 and 77.2

Image findings: the radiograph shows a fracture of the mid diaphysis (shaft) of the ulna. The fracture shows a break in one part of the cortex but the contralateral cortex of the ulna is intact. This is termed a 'greenstick' fracture where one side of the bone is broken and the other side bends but does not break.

Diagnosis: greenstick fracture.

Greenstick fractures occur in children due to the elasticity and pliability of their bones. They occur following an 'angulation' or 'bending' force, and involve the cortex on only one side of the bone, an incomplete fracture. There is associated angulation at the fracture site but this may only be subtle. In comparison, the bones of adults are far less pliable and a complete fracture involving both cortices is most likely to occur.

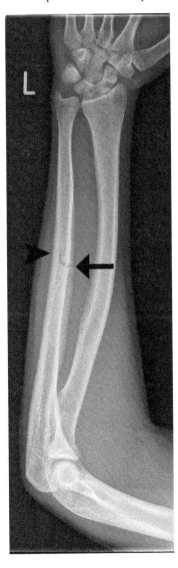

Figure 77.3 Plain radiograph of the forearm demonstrating a fracture line through the lateral ulnar cortex (arrow) and an intact medial cortex (arrowhead) in a patient with a greenstick fracture.

Children can, however, also have complete fractures as shown in Figures 77.4 and 77.5 which show a fracture line involving both cortices of the proximal ulna.

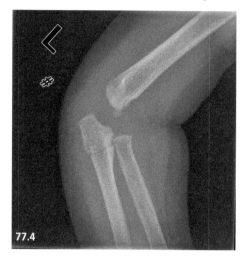

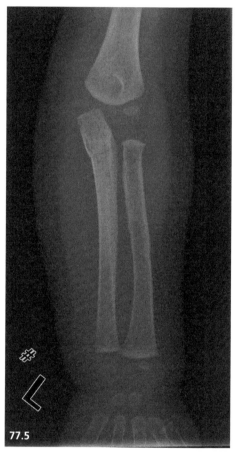

Figures 77.4 and 77.5

Case 78

A 32-year-old lady presented to her GP with a two-month history of feeling generally unwell. She had lost a stone in weight in the past month, and had recently been feeling feverish on and off, particularly at night when often she would wake up drenched with sweat. The GP requested for the following CXR to be performed.

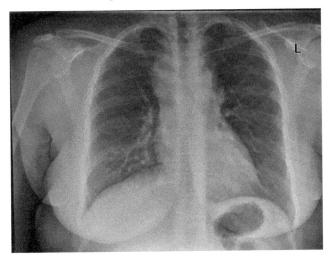

Figure 78.1

Image findings: the chest radiograph shows a widened superior mediastinum. This is particularly prominent in the right paratracheal region, with more lobulated soft tissue density seen lateral to the aortic knuckle on the left also.

A CT scan, *see* Figure 78.2, confirmed the cause of this mediastinal widening to be lymphandenopathy. Further enlarged nodes in the neck were biopsied and confirmed Hodgkin's lymphoma.

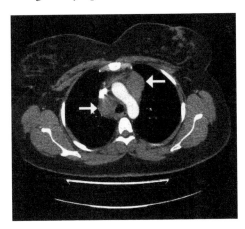

Figure 78.2 Contrast enhanced CT at the level of the aortic arch showing solid superior mediastinal masses in keeping with enlarged lymph nodes (arrows).

Diagnosis: Hodgkin's lymphoma.

The causes of a superior mediastinal mass on a chest radiograph are the 4 'T's:

- (terrible!) lymph nodes/lymphoma
- teratoma
- thymoma
- retrosternal thyroid extension.

CT is useful to differentiate which of these is the underlying cause.

Hodgkin's lymphoma arises in lymph nodes (90%), or the extranodal lymphoid tissues (10%) of the lung, gastrointestinal tract, or skin. Histologically the disease is characterised by the presence of Reed-Sternberg cells. It has a bimodal age distribution with peaks at 30 and 70 years of age. Patients often present with asymptomatic lymph node enlargement. The presence of 'B' symptoms (weight loss, fever, night sweats) is considered an unfavourable prognostic factor. Mediastinal nodes are involved in approximately 85% of cases at presentation (as in this case). Overall Hodgkin's lymphoma is one of the more curable forms of cancer, with survival rates of >90% when detected in the early stages. Treatment is with chemotherapy.

Non-Hodgkin's lymphoma is a group which includes all lymphomas that do not possess the Reed-Sternberg cell. These usually present in an older population >40 years. Presentation is usually through disease spread to the skin, lungs, bone or GI tract with ~65% having widespread disease at presentation. Lymphadenopathy is similarly more widespread and there is more likely to be infiltration of the liver and the spleen. Prognosis for non-Hodgkin's lymphoma is worse than for Hodgkin's.

Case 79

A 28-year-old male presented to accident and emergency at 2.30 a.m. He appeared intoxicated with alcohol. His friend gave the history that the patient had been involved in a fight outside a nightclub. He punched another man in the face. On examination the patient's right hand was bruised and swollen at the lateral aspect. The following radiographs were obtained.

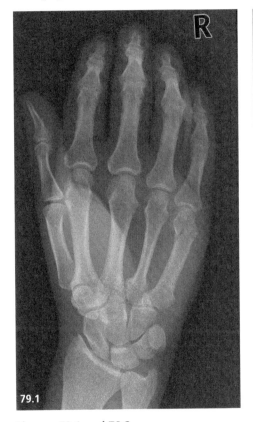 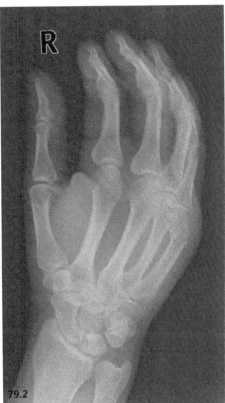

Figures 79.1 and 79.2

Image findings: AP and oblique radiographs of the right hand show a fracture through the neck of the fifth metacarpal.

Diagnosis: boxer's fracture.

Fifth (or fourth) metacarpal head fractures are otherwise known as a boxer's fracture (or fighter's/brawler's fracture). Typically they are caused by the impact of a clenched fist. The fractures are often angulated and may require reduction and pinning prior to splinting. In fact, boxers and others trained in punching (e.g. in the martial arts) are far less likely to sustain such an injury due to technique. When they do present with injury, it is often the second or third metacarpal which is fractured.

The second man who was involved in the fight also arrived in the emergency department complaining of right sided facial/eye pain. Figure 79.3 shows the facial radiograph obtained. This shows a fracture in the inferior wall of the right orbit with a fracture of the right zygoma. The most striking abnormality on the film is the difference in opacity of the maxillary sinuses. The maxillary sinus on the right is opacified and this is likely to be due to blood from the orbital fracture.

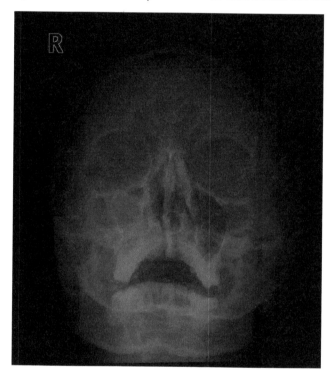

Figure 79.3 Facial view demonstrating a fracture of the inferior wall of the right orbit with opacification of the right maxillary antrum.

Case 80

A 66-year-old male had been found collapsed and unconscious on the floor at home by his wife when she returned home from shopping. Prior to her leaving the house he had been well. His past medical history included hypertension, for which he was on treatment. On arrival in accident and emergency the gentleman had a GCS of 9/15 with weakness down his left side. A CT head was requested to rule out intracranial pathology.

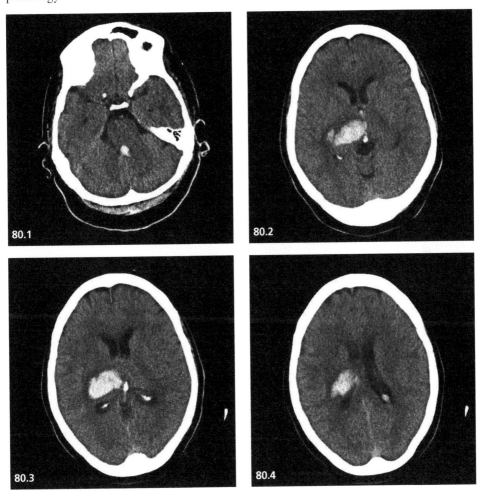

Figures 80.1, 80.2, 80.3 and 80.4

Image findings: the CT shows a large focus of high attenuation material (blood) within the basal ganglia region/thalamus on the right. There is also a trace of blood in the third ventricle (*see* Figure 80.2), and blood is filling (but not distending) the fourth ventricle (*see* Figure 80.1).

Diagnosis: intracerebral haemorrhage.

Approximately 10–15% of strokes are intracerebral bleeds while ~85% are ischaemic. There are several underlying causes for a haemorrhagic stroke rather than an ischaemic stroke which include:

- hypertension
- arterio-venous malformation (AVM)
- aneurysm
- coagulopathy
- drugs, e.g. anticoagulants.

Intracerebral bleeds can also occur as a consequence of trauma or there can be bleeding into an intracerebral tumour/metastasis.

CT is useful in the management of stroke since the main question to answer is – is the stroke due to ischaemia or haemorrhage? If the stroke is ischaemic then the patient would be treated with aspirin and may be a candidate for thrombolysis (if they presented within three hours of symptom onset to a stroke centre). If there is intracerebral haemorrhage then an assessment needs to be made regarding the resulting degree of mass effect. This is done by examining the CT to look for signs of midline shift and descent of the cerebellar tonsils. These are worrying signs since they indicate that there is a significant increase in intracerebral pressure and that the brain is being compressed. The only way the brain can expand is to extend through the foramen magnum which results in brainstem compression and can lead to death. These patients need urgent neurosurgical intervention and need to be considered for a procedure to evacuate the blood and relieve the pressure.

Case 81

A 50-year-old man presents to the emergency department in acute urinary retention. He reports a history of recurrent urinary tract infections with symptoms of frequency, nocturia and hesitancy. He also reports a long standing history of suprapubic pain. A kidneys-ureters-bladder (KUB) radiograph of the abdomen is requested.

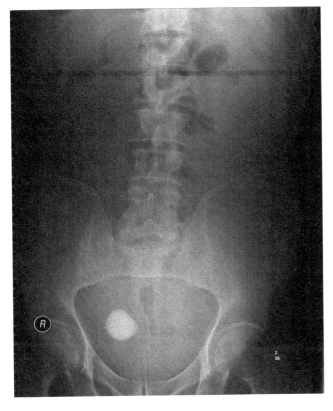

Figure 81.1

Image findings: there is a large calcified density projected over the right side of the pelvis. Appearances are consistent with a bladder calculus. No calculi are demonstrated in the kidneys or the ureters.

Diagnosis: large bladder calculus.

The most common cause of a bladder calculus is urinary stasis as a result of bladder outflow obstruction. A bladder calculus can also result from an anatomical abnormality of the urinary tract, a neurogenic bladder, infection or as a reaction to a foreign body. A bladder calculus may also originate from the kidneys before settling in the bladder. The majority of bladder calculi are non-radio-opaque and usually solitary.

Bladder calculi most frequently occur in men over the age of 50 with benign prostatic hypertrophy, as a result of urinary stasis due to the obstruction to the outflow of urine. Bladder calculi tend to be either composed of uric acid mixed with urate or a mixture of magnesium, ammonium and phosphate apatite.

An ultrasound is the ideal initial investigation to assess the urinary tract. A filled bladder is optimum to assess the bladder under ultrasound as it provides an acoustic window for the detection of abnormalities. Other radiological investigations available to assess the urinary tract include a KUB radiograph as in this case, an intravenous urogram (IVU) which has now been replaced by CT KUB in the majority of departments, and a CT urogram.

The medical management of bladder calculi involves attempting to dissolve the bladder calculi by urinary alkalinisation and correcting any contributing abnormalities in metabolism that may be present.

Surgical options for the treatment of bladder calculi include cystolitholapaxy, extracorporeal shock wave lithotripsy and cystolithotomy depending on the size of the calculus.

Case 82

A 50-year-old woman presents to her GP with a history of increasing shortness of breath over the last few months. She has a past medical history of bilateral mastectomies for breast cancer. A chest radiograph is requested.

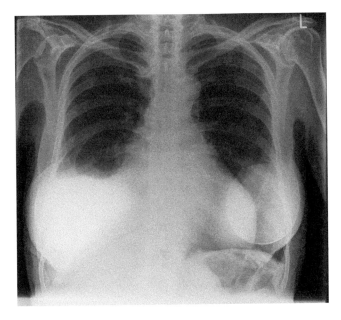

Figure 82.1

Image findings: this frontal chest radiograph demonstrates the presence of bilateral silicone breast implants. There is dense opacification in the right lower zone which forms a meniscus at its lateral edge. Appearances would be consistent with a moderate sized right pleural effusion.

Diagnosis: right-sided pleural effusion in a patient with bilateral silicone breast implants.

Breast cancers make up ~10% of the cancers in the world and are the second commonest cancer in women after lung cancer. Risk factors for breast cancer include age, sex, family history (BRCA gene), nulliparity, early menarche, late menopause and previous breast cancer. Breast cancer is usually either detected through self examination or through a breast cancer screening programme. In the UK all women aged 50–70 years are offered a three-yearly mammogram. Once detected, breast cancer is staged using the TNM staging system and treatment is offered depending on the spread of disease. Disease confined to a quadrant can be treated by wide local excision and radiotherapy. More diffuse disease within the breast may require a radical mastectomy and axillary lymph node clearance. If there is evidence of metastatic spread then chemotherapy and an oestrogen antagonist (tamoxifem) is used.

Approximately 20% of breast implants are used for reconstruction in breast cancer patients following mastectomy.

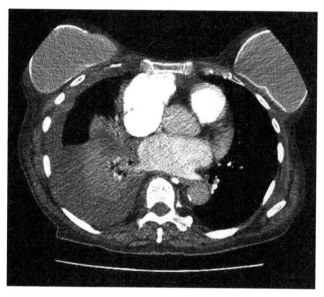

Figure 82.2

In this case, there is a moderate sized right pleural effusion, a CT scan of this patient is shown in Figure 82.2. The CT demonstrates the appearance of breast implants on CT. In this case the patient had undergone breast reconstruction surgery following bilateral mastectomies for breast carcinoma. In this context, the pleural effusion present on the chest radiograph and CT was highly suspicious for a malignant pleural effusion, an ultrasound guided diagnostic tap was performed which confirmed the diagnosis. Common sites for breast metastases are:

- axillary lymph nodes
- bone – lytic or sclerotic metastases
- liver
- lungs.

Case 83

A 68-year-old man presented to his GP with six-month history of weight loss. He was a smoker – smoking 30 cigarettes a day for more than 45 years. He had had a few episodes of haemoptysis over the last three months and was feeling generally unwell. He had a previous history of a myocardial infarction five years ago and suffered with type 2 diabetes. A CXR was requested.

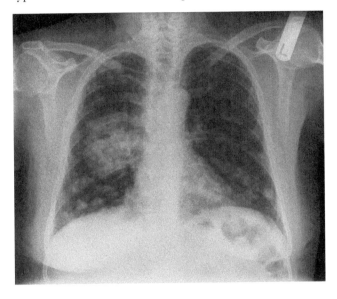

Figure 83.1

Image findings: the chest radiograph shows a large solid 7 cm mass lesion in the right mid zone. There are multiple smaller nodules seen throughout both lungs. Appearances would be highly suspicious for a primary bronchogenic cancer with multiple lung metastases.

The patient was urgently referred for a rapid access lung cancer hospital appointment and a subsequent CT chest was performed.

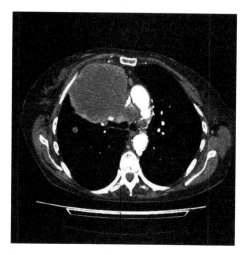

Figure 83.2 Axial CT image showing a large necrotic tumour in the right middle lobe invading the mediastinum due to primary bronchogenic carcinoma.

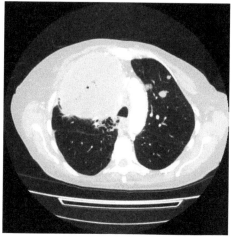

Figure 83.3 Axial CT image on lung windows shows lung nodules in the left lung.

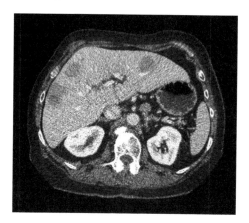

Figure 83.4 Axial CT image showing liver metastases.

The axial CT images show a large mass filling the anterior right hemithorax and invading the mediastinum. The mass lesion appears to have a low attenuation more fluid centre, which is due to central necrosis. On the lung window images there are some small locules of gas within the lesion and this is because the patient had just had a lung biopsy. Small well defined nodules in the left upper lobe are due to lung metastases. CT image from the upper abdomen, *see* Figure 83.4, also shows several lesions within the liver consistent with liver metastases.

Diagnosis: lung cancer.

Lung cancer is the commonest cancer in men worldwide and is the leading cause of cancer death in men (~35% of all cancer deaths). Presentation is with cough, haemoptysis, weight loss and chest pain though sometimes the cancer can be an incidental finding on a chest radiograph being performed for some other region. Lung cancer is classified according to the histological subtype:

- adenocarcinoma (50%) – commoner in women and non-smokers. Usually peripheral in position
- squamous cell carcinoma (35%) – strong association with smoking. Two thirds central in location. Central necrosis and cavitation is common
- small cell carcinoma (15%) – strong association with smoking. Highly likely to metastasise. Usually central and is the most likely to cause superior vena cava obstruction
- large cell carcinoma (<5%) – strong association with smoking. Usually peripheral and bulky mass.

Bronchogenic carcinomas usually spread to the lung, mediastinal and hilar lymph nodes, liver, adrenals and bone. They can also present with paraneoplastic syndromes, e.g. Cushing syndrome, syndrome of inappropriate antidiuretic hormone secretion (SIADH). Treatment of lung cancer is dependent on accurate staging of the tumour. This is done using CT to determine the TNM staging. Where there is uncertainty about nodal involvement then PET/CT and lymph node biopsy either using surgical cervical mediastinoscopy/nodal sampling or endobronchial ultrasound biopsy (EBUS) is used.

TNM staging:

- T1a – tumour size <2 cm
- T1b – tumour size 2–3 cm
- T2a – tumour size 3–5 cm
- T2b – tumour size 5–7 cm
- T3 – tumour size >7 cm; chest wall/pericardium/diaphragm invasion; collapse/obstructive pneumonitis of the whole lung/satellite nodules in the same lobe
- T4 – mediastinal invasion/satellite nodules in other ipsilateral lobes
- N1-3 nodal involvement on ipsilateral (N1)/central (N2)/contralateral (N3) sides of the mediastinum
- M0 – no metastasis
- M1a – tumour nodules in the contralateral lung/pleural nodules/malignant pleural effusion
- M1b – distant metastases.

Localised disease is amenable to surgical resection whilst more diffuse or invasive disease requires chemotherapy/radiotherapy.

Case 84

An 81-year-old female presented to her GP feeling generally unwell with a six-month history of weight loss. More recently her husband had noticed a drooping of her right eyelid and had insisted she visit the GP. She had been a smoker for the last 60 years. On examination the GP confirmed a right ptosis and also noted that the right pupil was constricted. The GP requested a CXR.

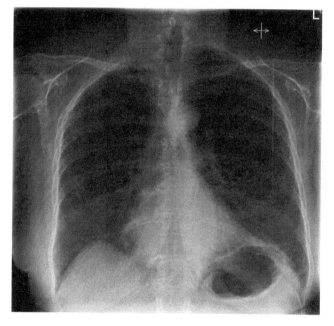

Figure 84.1

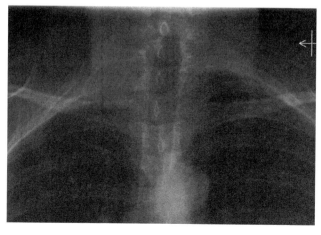

Figure 84.2

Image findings: the chest radiograph shows a soft tissue opacity in the right lung apex. The posterior aspect of the right second rib is not visible and has been destroyed. Findings were confirmed on CT, *see* Figure 84.3. Appearances would therefore be of a right pancoast tumour.

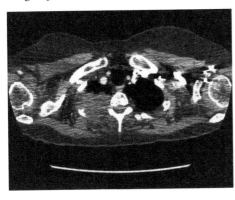

Figure 84.3

Diagnosis: right pancoast tumour (superior sulcus tumour).

Mass lesions in the lung apices are often overlooked and it is important that the lung apices are consciously reviewed on every CXR. They are collectively called Pancoast tumours (named after the US radiologist Henry Pancoast who first described them in 1924). Pancoast tumours account for 3% of lung cancers. These tumour masses are usually squamous cell carcinomas. Staging and treatment is as for lung cancers in other positions (*see* Case 83).

Due to the relatively confined space in which they arise, they often present with symptoms relating to direct invasion of adjacent structures:

- arm pain is common due to brachial plexus involvement
- Horner's syndrome (a triad of partial ptosis, unilateral papillary constriction (meiosis), and loss of sweating on the same side of the face (anhydrosis) occurs due to involvement of the sympathetic chain
- shoulder and rib pain from local bony destruction (this can often be identified on the CXR, as long as it is looked for)!

Case 85

A 65-year-old lady with a large soft tissue mass in the right lung was referred for a PET/CT scan for staging. She had already undergone CT guided biopsy of the lesion, which confirmed adenocarcinoma.

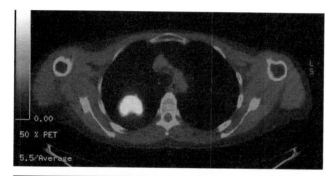

Figure 85.1

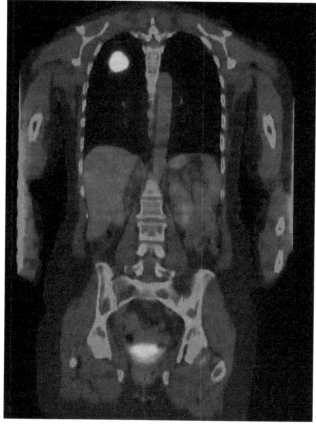

Figure 85.2

Image findings: the selected images are from the PET/CT – Figure 85.1 is an axial fused PET/CT image and Figure 85.2 is a coronal reconstruction fused PET/CT image demonstrating the right upper lobe mass which shows marked metabolic activity (it looks 'hot'). Further activity is seen in the kidneys and bladder on the coronal reconstruction (this is normal as the tracer is excreted via the kidneys). No further significant increased metabolic activity was demonstrated on this examination. In particular, there was no uptake in the mediastinal lymph nodes.

Diagnosis: lung cancer with no mediastinal nodal involvement.

Positron emission tomography (PET) is a nuclear medicine technique that uses positron emitting radioisotopes with short half lives. The commonest isotope used in clinical work is Fluorine-18, which has a half life of 109 minutes. This is produced in a cyclotron. The radioisotope is incorporated into a biologically active glucose analogue called FDG (2-[fluorine-18]fluoro-2 deoxy-D-glucose). This glucose analogue is then injected into the patient where it concentrates in the most metabolically active cells within the body. Tumour cells with a high mitotic rate are highly metabolically active and will therefore take up the tracer. To minimise metabolic activity elsewhere in the body the patient is starved for six hours prior to the test (to limit GI tract activity), and strenuous exercise is avoided for the prior 24 hours (to limit muscle uptake). Also the patient is encouraged not to talk after the injection to minimise uptake in muscles of the head and neck (especially when being assessed for head and neck tumours).

The scan will be performed approximately one hour after injection. As the name suggests, the radioisotope decays by the emission of positrons. The emitted positron will almost immediately collide with an electron in an event called annihilation. This produces two gamma-ray photons which move apart in opposite directions. These are high energy photons that then easily pass through the body and are detected by the scanner. The technique relies on simultaneous (coincident) detection of both photons. Any single pulses due to background radiation are ignored by the system electronics.

The PET scan produces a 'map' of metabolic activity. A non-contrast CT scan is then performed in order to provide anatomical information and the two scans are then fused to give the final PET/CT images shown in this example.

In this case of known adenocarcinomas of the lung, the PET scan has been performed to assess the stage of the disease. The CT chest suggested that some mediastinal nodes may possibly be involved but PET/CT was requested to check this. In this case no further disease was found and the patient was able to undergo potentially curable surgery.

PET/CT is currently used in the UK for staging in:

- lung cancer
- oesophageal cancer
- head and neck cancers
- lymphoma.

But can also be used for:

- differentiating between benign and malignant lesions
- identifying cancer recurrence
- assessing response to cancer treatment
- differentiating post surgical scarring from residual/recurrent disease.

Case 86

A 24-year-old girl had been referred to gastroenterology outpatient clinic by her GP. She had recently arrived in the country from Russia and spoke very little English. Unfortunately she had no legible medical notes, but via a translator the GP had managed to ascertain she had long standing problems with her bowel. On examination the patient had a small sinus in the skin in the right iliac fossa, which was draining liquid faeculant material into a bag. She also had a history of abdominal pain, diarrhoea, and weight loss, worse over the past few months. On examination there was generalised abdominal tenderness, worse in the right iliac fossa. There were also perianal skin tags and a few oral aphthous ulcers. The gastroenterologist felt sure of the diagnosis and organised a barium follow-through examination as one of his investigations.

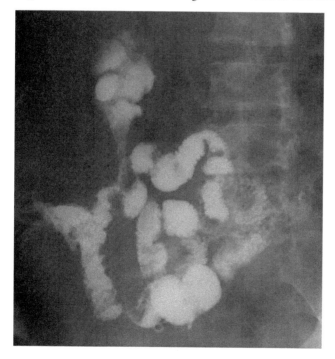

Figure 86.1

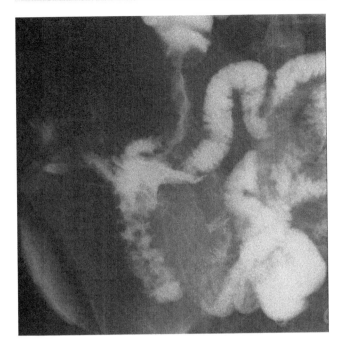

Figure 86.2

Image findings: the selected images are from a barium follow through examination. The images show marked abnormality of the terminal and distal ileum with stricturing and a cobblestone pattern of ulceration. A sinus tract can be seen extending from the terminal ileum to the skin surface, with contrast draining into the bag.

Diagnosis: Crohn's disease.

Crohn's disease is an inflammatory process that can involve the entire length of the GI tract from mouth to anus. Typically the small bowel is affected, and in particular the terminal ileum. The disease is often found at multiple sites, with relatively normal bowel in between ('skip-lesions'). Deep ('rose-thorn') ulcers and fissures in the mucosa are characteristic, forming a 'cobblestone' appearance. Pathologically it is characterised by transmural inflammation. It usually has symptom onset in the second to fourth decades.

Complications of Crohn's disease include:

- fistulae – seen in up to one third of cases. Fistulae can be enterocolic (bowel to bowel), enterocutaneous (bowel to skin – as in this case); enterovesical (bowel to bladder) or perianal
- abscess development
- perforation
- obstruction due to stricturing
- slight increased risk of developing colorectal cancer
- increased risk of developing small and large bowel lymphoma.

Crohn's disease can also have many extraintestinal manifestations such as an association with gallstones, fatty liver, renal stones, ankylosing spondylitis, uveitis and erythema nodosum. Treatment is usually by steroids and immunosuppressants. Surgical intervention is usually required when complications arise.

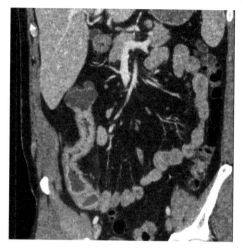

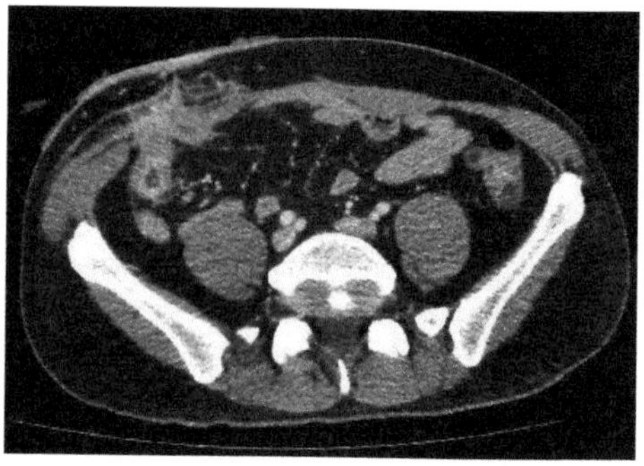

Figure 86.4 Axial CT images in the same patient demonstrating the inflammation around a thickened terminal ileum which is forming an enterocutaneous fistula.

Figure 86.3 Coronal reconstruction showing the terminal ileal stricture in a patient with Crohn's disease.

Crohn's can usually be differentiated from the other commonest inflammatory bowel condition – ulcerative colitis (UC). UC is an idiopathic inflammatory bowel syndrome which always involves the rectum extending more proximally. Disease is continuous with no skip lesions and is usually confined to the large bowel (though some 5% of patients can get a backwash ileitis). Disease is confined to the mucosa/submucosa and is not transmural. It is characterised by shallow mucosal ulcers and inflammatory pseudopolyps. In the chronic stages a 'lead pipe' colon develops which is rigid and narrowed. It usually has two peaks of onset in the third to fifth decades and the seventh to eighth. It is complicated by toxic megacolon, perforation, strictures and a significantly increased risk of colonic adenocarcinoma. Fistulation is not a feature.

Case 87

A 25-year-old lady complains of numbness of the right side of her face, which eventually resolves. Subsequently she complains of numbness of the left side of her face and left arm. Neurological examination is normal. An MRI brain and cervical spine is requested to rule out any underlying pathology.

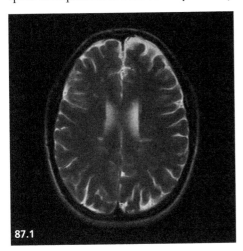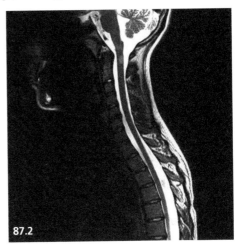

Figures 87.1 and 87.2

Image findings: Figure 87.1 is a T2 weighted MRI scan of the brain (CSF appears bright on T2 weighted imaging, therefore the ventricles appear bright). There are multiple ovoid high signal (bright) lesions in the white matter of the brain, orientated perpendicular to the ventricle wall.

Figure 87.2 is a T2 weighted MRI scan of the cervical spine in the same patient (the CSF around the cord appears bright). This demonstrates two ovoid high signal lesions in the cord at the level of the craniocervical junction and at the C1/C2 level. This is a case of multiple sclerosis (MS), with lesions present in the brain and cervical spine.

Diagnosis: multiple sclerosis.

Multiple sclerosis (MS) is a chronic inflammatory disease characterised by a relapsing and remitting course. Plaques of demyelination occur throughout the CNS. The aetiology is unclear and diagnosis is primarily clinical – with a history of recurrent episodes of neurological symptoms attributed to more than one part of the CNS. Tests include CSF electrophoresis which is positive for oligoclonal bands.

CT may be normal, or show periventricular isoattenuating (same density as brain parencyhyma) or hypoattenuating (darker density than brain parenchyma) lesions. There may be transient enhancement of lesions with contrast in the acute stage.

MRI is the investigation of choice for suspected MS. Lesions can occur anywhere in the central nervous system, including the brainstem, cerebellum, corpus callosum and optic tract. However, lesions are commonest in the periventricular white matter.

MRI findings:

- typically, ovoid lesions are seen with their long axis orientated perpendicular to the ventricular walls (due to perivenous demyelination) These lesions are also known as 'Dawson fingers'. Although periventricular lesions are very suggestive of MS, these lesions are non-specific and must be correlated with clinical picture. MS lesions are high signal (bright) on T2 weighted imaging and fluid attenuated inversion recovery (FLAIR)
- the spinal cord is commonly involved, particularly the cervical cord. The plaques are orientated along the spinal cord axis
- there may be enhancement of lesions, usually peripherally
- there may be cerebral atrophy in chronic MS. The ventricles may be enlarged and the sulci prominent.

Case 88

A 22-year-old man who had sustained head trauma three weeks previously presents with collapse and a seizure. On examination, there is a discharging wound over his forehead. He is not known to have epilepsy. A CT head is performed.

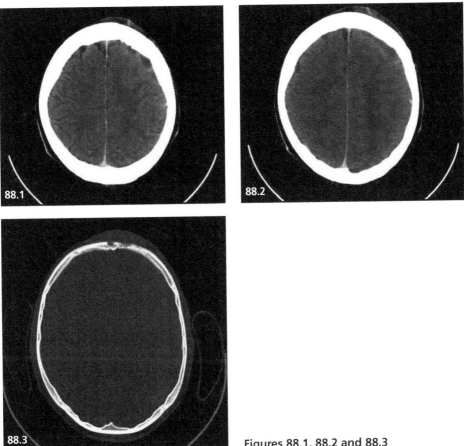

Figures 88.1, 88.2 and 88.3

Image findings: Figure 88.1 is a non-enhanced CT of the brain demonstrating a subtle low density (dark) extra-axial (within the skull but outside of the brain) collection along the convexity in the left frontal region. Appearances are suspicious of an abscess, so intravenous contrast was administered.

Figure 88.2 is a CT brain performed with contrast demonstrating rim enhancement of the collection, which is crescenteric in shape. This man has a subdural empyema/abscess. In this case, the subdural empyema/abscess was due to calvarial osteomyelitis.

Figure 88.3 is the CT brain of the same patient on bony windows demonstrating bony destruction of the skull due to osteomyelitis.

Diagnosis: subdural empyema/abscess.

A subdural empyema is a loculated collection of pus in the subdural space. Pus may also extend into the epidural space. Subdural empyemas (like subdural haematomas) are commonly found along the convexity of the brain adjacent to the inner table and are typically crescenteric in shape. Epidural empyemas are typically biconvex in shape. The collection is usually isodense (same density as CSF) or hypodense on non-contrast enhanced CT. Contrast enhanced CT demonstrates rim enhancement of the collection.

In contrast, a cerebral abscess is infection of the brain parenchyma. It occurs typically at the grey-white matter junction in the frontal and temporal lobes. CT demonstrates a low density lesion (dark) with an enhancing capsule. In the early stages, the capsule is typically thin. In the later stages, the capsule may thicken and become multiloculated and 'daughter' abscesses may appear.

Occasionally, in infants and young children, subdural effusions associated with meningitis may become infected producing an empyema. In older children and adults, subdural empyemas may be associated with paranasal sinusitis, otitis media, infection after craniotomy or a penetrating wound. Differential diagnoses include subacute or chronic subdural haematoma and subdural effusion.

Subdural empyemas are considered a neurosurgical emergency and an urgent opinion must be obtained.

Case 89

A 50-year-old woman has a chest X-ray performed for chronic cough and dyspnoea. She has been a smoker for the last 30 years.

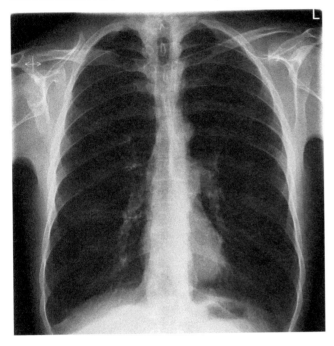

Figure 89.1

Image findings: Figure 89.1 shows hyperinflation of the lungs. There are almost nine anterior ribs visualised in the mid clavicular line. The hemidiaphragms are also flattened. This is a chest X-ray showing changes of emphysema.

Diagnosis: emphysema.

In emphysema there is destruction of alveolar walls, *see* Figure 89.2, leading to permanently enlarged air spaces distal to the terminal bronchiole.

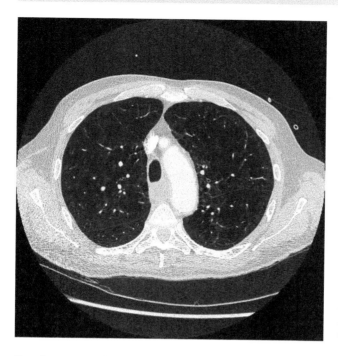

Figure 89.2 Axial CT image on lung windows shows destruction of the alveolar walls with large air spaces.

Emphysema is a disease of smokers with 40–50% developing emphysema. Coal workers are also at risk of developing emphysema. In these cases the emphysematous changes are usually worse in the upper lobes/apices. An enzyme deficiency – Alpha-1-antitrypsin – can result in emphysema in young patients with distribution predominantly in the lung bases. The imaging findings are of:

- hyperinflation of the chest – characterised by flattening of the hemidiaphragms, long, thin appearance of the heart shadow due to overinflation/low diaphragms
- abnormal pulmonary vasculature – emphysema has an uneven distribution and there is usually reduction is size of vessels in affected areas particularly in the lung periphery
- bullae – large air filled spaces develop more commonly at the apices.

The distribution of alveolar wall destruction can either cause centrilobular emphysema (central) or paraseptal (peripheral and subpleural) or a mixture of both.

Spirometry demonstrates an obstructive pattern. Treatment is aimed at stopping smoking, bronchodilators and steroids/antibiotics to treat acute exacerbations. As emphysema gets progressively worse it can lead to pulmonary hypertension and right heart failure (cor pulmonale).

Chronic obstructive pulmonary disease (COPD) encompasses asthma, chronic bronchitis, and emphysema.

Case 90

A 63-year-old female presents with left-sided loin to groin pain. A plain film of the kidneys, ureters and bladder (KUB) is performed.

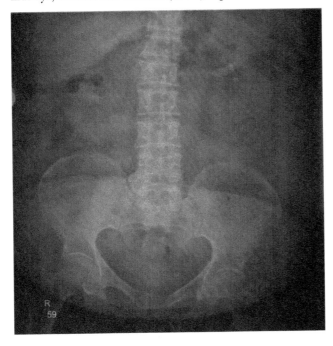

Figure 90.1

Image findings: there is an irregular dense calcific opacity projected over the left kidney. This patient has a partial staghorn calculus, *see* Figure 90.2

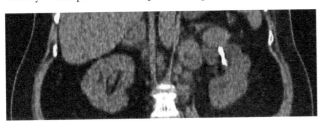

Figure 90.2 Coronal multi-planar reformat CT in the same patient demonstrating the staghorn calculus in the mid and upper pole of the left kidney.

Diagnosis: renal calculus.

Renal calculi are due to crystal aggregations formed when the urine becomes supersaturated with a salt. Renal calculi may be asymptomatic. Stones obstructing the ureteropelvic junction may present with flank pain (due to distension of the renal capsule). Stones in the ureter may cause colicky pain radiating from the loin to groin, associated with nausea and vomiting.

Approximately 80% to 90% of renal calculi are visible on plain film. Contrast this with gallstones where 15% to 20% are calcified and radio-opaque on plain film.

There are four basic chemical types of renal calculi:

1   calcium – the majority of these are composed of calcium oxalate (75%)
2   struvite – magnesium ammonium phosphate (struvite) stones are the second commonest stone (15%) and are the most common constituent of staghorn calculus. A staghorn calculus is a branched calculus filling the entire bifid renal collecting system. They form with recurrent urinary tract infections
3   uric acid – (5%)
4   cystine – cystine stones (1% to 2%) are mildly radio-opaque and are found in patients with congenital cystinuria.

Although most calculi are radio-opaque on plain film, differentiation from other causes of abdominal calcifications, such as phleboliths limits the accuracy of plain film. Intravenous urogram is being superseded by non-contrast CT. CT of the kidneys, ureters and bladder (CT KUB) is considered the gold standard for detecting urinary tract calculi. Ultrasound is less sensitive than CT for the detection of renal calculi, but can demonstrate the presence of hydronephrosis and is also useful in pregnant patients. Ultrasound will show a highly echogenic (bright) focus with posterior acoustic shadowing.

Case 91

An 88-year-old gentleman has a plain abdominal radiograph taken for abdominal pain, vomiting and constipation.

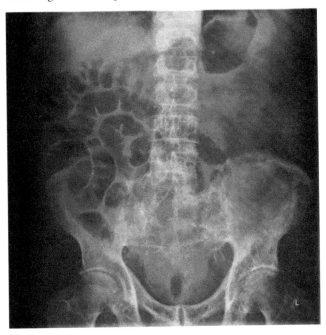

Figure 91.1

Image findings: the plain abdominal film shows several prominent small bowel loops, but no evidence of bowel obstruction. However, incidentally, there is bony expansion, trabecular coarsening and cortical thickening of the left hemi-pelvis. This patient has Paget's disease of the pelvis.

Diagnosis: Paget's disease of bone.

Paget's disease of bone is characterised by excessive bone remodelling. There is increased resorption of bone (due to an increased number of osteoclasts) and increased formation of bone (due to an increased number of osteoblasts). Newly formed bone is abnormally soft with a disorganised trabecular pattern.

The disease is rare below the age of 40 and more common in Caucasians. Individuals affected may be asymptomatic or present with a variety of symptoms including fatigue, hearing loss, blindness, facial nerve palsy, and pain. The pelvis is affected in 75%. Other areas commonly involved are the lumbar spine, thoracic spine, proximal femur and calvarium. Alkaline phosphatase is usually significantly elevated. The disease may be divided into three stages.

1 **Active phase (osteolytic):** this phase may predominate early in the disease and is characterised by aggressive bone resorption.
   - Osteoporosis circumscripta of skull (well-defined lysis of the outer table of the skull).
   - Flame-shaped radiolucencies at the ends of long bones.
2 **Mixed lytic and sclerotic phase:** this phase is common. There is decreased osteoclastic activity and increased osteoblastic activity.
   - There is coexistence of lytic and sclerotic phases, e.g. in the skull – osteoporosis circumscripta with focal areas of bone sclerosis. In the pelvis – mixed osteolytic and osteosclerotic areas.
3 **Inactive phase (osteosclerotic):** there is decreased osteoblastic activity with decreased bone turnover.
   - Thickening of the skull vault with 'cotton wool' areas of sclerotic bone.
   - In the spine, there is thickening of the vertebral cortex producing a classic 'picture frame' appearance. 'Ivory' vertebra describes the increased density of vertebra.

Complications of Paget's disease include, pathological fracture, malignant change (osteosarcoma), neurological complications such as nerve entrapment and spinal stenosis, early onset osteoarthritis and high output congestive cardiac failure.

Case 92

A 20-year-old man presents to his GP with right lower leg pain and swelling which has been getting worse over the last few weeks. Radiographs of the lower leg are requested.

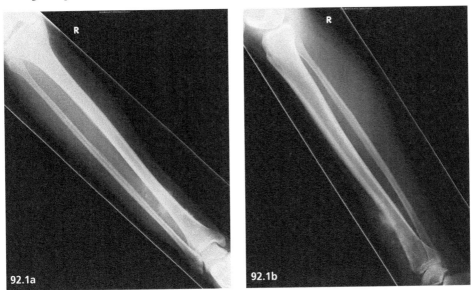

Figure 92.1a, b

Image findings: these images are AP and lateral views of the right distal tibia and fibula. There is an aggressive periosteal reaction along the diaphysis of the distal tibia with short spicules of new bone perpendicular to the shaft of the tibia (sunburst pattern). There is cortical thickening but no evidence of cortical destruction.

Diagnosis: osteosarcoma.

Osteosarcoma is the second most common primary malignant bone tumour after multiple myeloma. The peak incidence of osteosarcoma occurs in the second decade. There are several types of osteosarcomas with each type having distinctive clinical, radiological and histological characteristics. The most common type is the conventional osteosarcoma (75%) which usually has an associated soft tissue mass. A conventional osteosarcoma has a radiographic appearance of a poorly defined intramedullary mass that extends through the cortex. Other types of osteosarcoma include telangiectatic osteosarcoma, parosteal/periosteal osteosarcoma, multicentric osteosarcoma, gnathic osteosarcoma and secondary osteosarcoma (arise in pre-existing bone lesions such as Paget's). Osteosarcomas commonly occur at sites of high skeletal growth such as the metaphyseal regions of the distal femur, proximal tibia and proximal humerus.

A plain radiograph is the usual first line investigation to evaluate a bony lesion, particularly the degree of bone destruction and periosteal reaction. Osteosarcomas can have variable appearance of the plain film, the following is a list of the common radiographic findings in osteosarcoma:

- moth-eaten pattern of bone destruction
- aggressive periosteal reaction such as a sunburst pattern or codmans triangle (raised periosteum)
- poorly defined intramedullary mass that extends through the cortex.
- associated soft tissue mass
- sclerotic/lytic/mixed sclerotic lytic bone lesions.

MRI helps to evaluate the extent of tumour infiltration within the bone marrow and soft tissue, as well as the relationship of the tumour to adjacent vessels and nerves for surgical planning, *see* Figures 92.2 a and b. Osteosarcomas are aggressive tumours, treatment involves surgical resection of the tumour with a wide resection margin and chemotherapy. Amputation may be necessary depending on the size and site of the osteosarcoma.

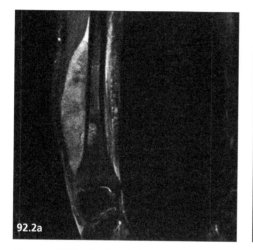
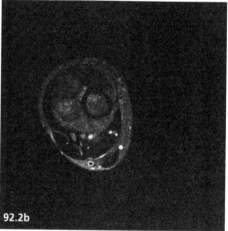

Figures 92.2a, b T2 weighted MRI image of the tibia shows a poorly defined bone lesion with a significant soft tissue component.

Case 93

A 50-year-old woman is seen by her GP complaining of painful and stiff hands worse in the mornings. On examination her wrist and hands are warm and swollen with ulnar deviation of the metacarpophalangeal joints. She reports having had previous hand surgery. Plain radiographs of the hands are requested.

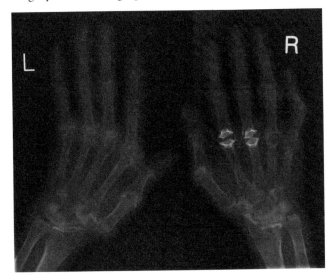

Figure 93.1

Image findings: there is a symmetrical polyarticular arthropathy predominantly affecting the metacarpophalangeal (MCP) joints and carpal joints. There is joint space narrowing, fusion of the carpal bones, central erosions and generalised osteopaenia of the affected joints. There is ulnar deviation at the MCP joints with joint replacements of the right second and third MCP joints. Appearances are consistent with rheumatoid arthritis (RA) of the wrist and hands.

Diagnosis: rheumatoid arthritis.

RA is a systemic inflammatory disease characterised by inflammation and destruction of synovial joints and bone which leads to joint deformity and loss of function. RA has a female preponderance with a female to male ratio of 3:1. RA is a symmetrical polyarticular arthopathy of an insidious onset typically affecting the small joints of the hands and feet, *see* Figure 93.2 with intermittent 'flare-ups'. Patients commonly present with morning stiffness lasting more than an hour, multiple painful and swollen joints and fatigue. There will be 85% of patients with a positive serum rheumatoid factor. RA is a systemic disease and is associated with a number of extra-articular manifestations including Felty syndrome, Sjögren syndrome, RA vasculitis, pericarditis and rheumatoid lung nodules.

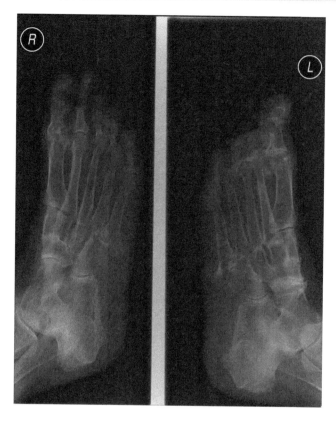

Figure 93.2 Oblique images of both feet show classical features of rheumatoid arthritis with erosions at the bases of the metatarsals and the metatarsophalangeal joints; periarticular osteopaenia and deformity of the joints.

Examination of rheumatoid hands frequently reveals joint swelling, tenderness to palpation, joint deformity and pain on active or passive movement of affected joints.

A plain radiograph of the affected joint remains the first line investigation to assess the severity of RA. MRI has the ability to detect early joint disease and provide detailed joint anatomy if surgical intervention is being considered. Ultrasound is also a useful adjunct for the assessment of specific joints and guide steroid joint injections.

Common findings seen on a plain radiograph of a rheumatoid hand include:

- periarticular soft tissue swelling
- juxta-articular osteopaenia
- joint space narrowing
- marginal and central bone erosions
- Swan neck and boutonnière deformity of the interphalangeal joints.
- joint subluxation and fusion.

Medical options for the management of RA include analagesia, NSAIDs, prednisolone and disease modifying antirheumatic drugs such as methotrexate – depending on the severity of the disease. Surgical options include joint replacement, intra-articular drug injections and joint fusion.

Case 94

A 64-year-old lady attended her local breast screening service following a routine recall invitation. She has no breast symptoms, and all previous screening visits have been normal. Below are the standard two mammographic views (cranio-caudal (CC), and mediolateral-oblique (MLO) of each breast.

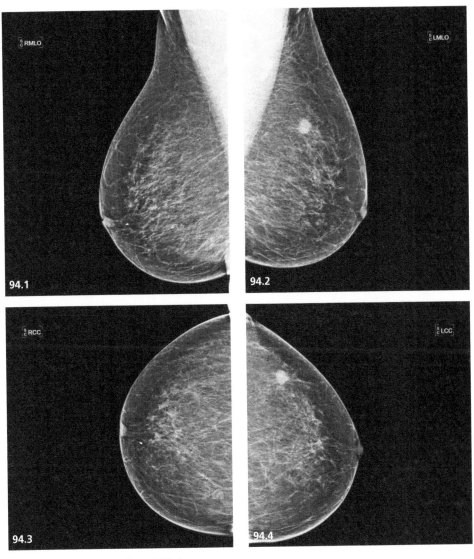

Figures 94.1, 94.2, 94.3 and 94.4

Image findings: the mammograms show a small (approximately 1.5 cm) dense opacity in the upper outer quadrant of the left breast. Its outer margin is spiculated. This is a breast carcinoma.

Diagnosis: breast cancer.

The NHS National Breast Screening Programme provides free breast screening every three years for all women between the ages of 50 and 70 years. By 2012 this will expand to ages 47 to 73 years. The aim of the screening programme is to detect the cancer at an earlier stage when it is more treatable.

If an abnormality is detected on the screening mammogram the patient will be recalled to the assessment clinic for further investigations. These may include clinical examination, more mammograms at different angles, and ultrasound scan of the breast. A sample of the tissue is then needed for definitive diagnosis. This is usually obtained by percutaneous core biopsy using ultrasound or stereotactic X-ray guidance.

Contrast enhanced MRI can also be used to determine whether the disease is focally located within a single quadrant (in which case, may be amenable to a wide local excision) or whether there is multifocal disease (radical mastectomy would need to be considered).

Routine mammography is also offered to younger patients where there is a strong family history of breast cancer. Genetic studies can be done in these patients to determine whether or not they carry a mutated BRCA 1 or 2 gene which carries a significantly higher risk of developing breast cancer. Approximately 10–12% of women in the general population will develop breast cancer in their lifetime, which increases to ~60% of women who carry the mutated BRCA1 or 2 gene. So, this carries a 5–6 times increased risk. Women who carry the gene can elect to have surveillance follow up with imaging/clinical input or can elect to have prophylactic surgery.

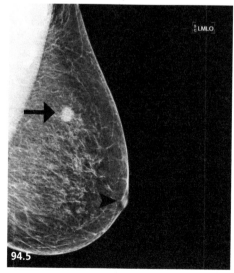 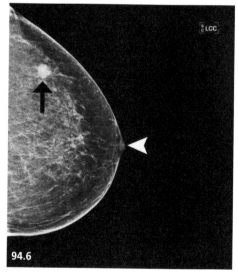

Figures 94.5 and 94.6 Spiculated mass (arrow) in the left breast. The position of the mass within the breast tissue is determined by identification of the nipple (arrowhead), and knowing which are the medial, lateral, superior and inferior borders of the breast on the standard views.

Case 95

A 12-year-old boy is taken to his GP after his mother feels a non-tender bony lump around the child's knee. A plain radiograph of both the knees is requested.

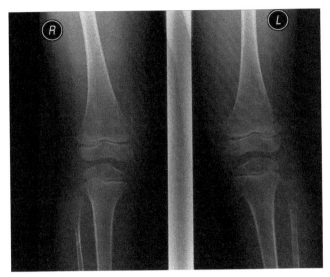

Figure 95.1

Image findings: this is an AP view of both knees. There are a few pedunculated bony exostoses pointing away from the knee joint. The cortices of the bony lesions are in continuation with the host bone. In the left knee there is also a sessile broad based bony exostosis at the medial aspect of the tibial metaphysis pointing away from the tibial epiphysis. There is no evidence of bony destruction. The overall appearances are consistent with multiple osteochondromata.

Diagnosis: hereditary multiple exostoses.

A solitary osteochondroma is the most common benign bone lesion and is usually diagnosed between the first and third decade of life. An osteochondroma is a cartilage covered bony exostosis that arises from the bone surface. It usually presents as a non-tender painless mass near a joint, commonly at the metaphysis of a long bone such as the femur and tibia. Occasionally an osteochondroma can present with symptoms such as numbness and tingling as a result of pressure on adjacent nerves or blood vessels.

    A plain radiograph is usually the only imaging study required as an osteochondroma has a characteristic appearance. Osteochondromas appear as pedunculated or sessile bony lesions with well-defined margins. The cortex of the lesion appears in continuation with the cortex of the host bone, as does the medullary component. In addition, osteochondromas typically point away from the nearest joint.

Hereditary multiple exostoses (HME) is a condition characterised by the presence of multiple osteochondromas, *see* Figures 95.1 and 95.2. It is also commonly known as multiple hereditary osteochondromata, familial osteochondromatosis and diaphyseal aclasia. It is a hereditary, autosomal-dominant disorder with incomplete penetrance in females. There is an increased risk of malignant transformation in multiple hereditary osteochondromata (5%) compared to a solitary osteochondroma (1%). In addition to multiple osteochondromas, other radiological findings seen in HME include disproportionate shortening of an extremity (50%), pseudo-Madelung deformity (Figure 95.2) and Erlenmeyer flask deformity.

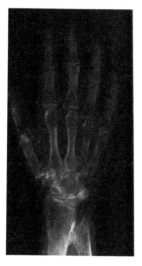 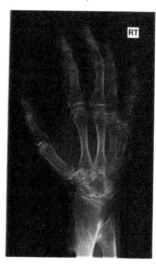

Figure 95.2 Images of the wrist demonstrate a pseudo-Madelung deformity which is characterised by shortening of the ulna with a long bowed radius and ulnar angulation of the distal radial articular surface.

Osteochondromas do not usually require any treatment and can be routinely followed up. Surgical resection however is indicated if the diagnosis is uncertain, if the lesion becomes painful or the lesion causes symptoms from compression of adjacent nerves and vessels.

Case 96

A 78-year-old lady was brought to accident and emergency complaining of pain and swelling in the right hip and thigh. This had been getting worse over the past 24 hours, and she was now also feeling very unwell and feverish. She denied any history of fall or trauma to the hip, but had been unable to weight bear today. She is a known diabetic. On examination she appeared unwell, febrile and tachycardic. Any movement of the right hip worsened the pain. The right thigh appeared hot, swollen and erythematous, and was tender to touch. The white cell count and CRP were raised on the initial bloods and an initial diagnosis of cellulitis was made. The surgical team were called. The following radiographs of the right hip were requested to exclude a bony injury.

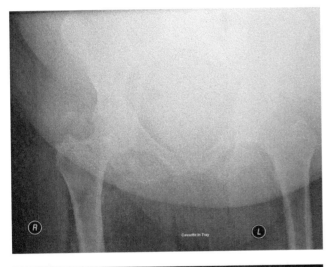

Figure 96.1

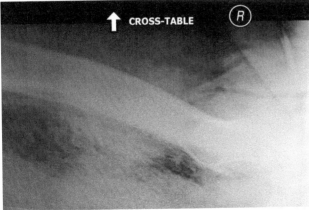

Figure 96.2

Image findings: the radiographs show an extensive amount of air/gas within the soft tissues of the upper right thigh. This is in keeping with necrotising fasciitis. A CT was requested prior to theatre to further define the extent of disease.

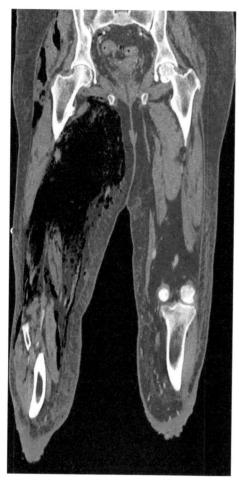

Figure 96.3 Coronal reconstruction CT image clearly demonstrates the extent of the gas within the medial and posterior compartments of the right thigh.

Diagnosis: necrotising fasciitis.

Necrotising fasciitis is a rapidly spreading soft tissue infection. It occurs in the deep fascial layers, and results in secondary necrosis of the subcutaneous tissues. The infection is characterised by the presence of gas forming organisms and consequently air is seen within the subcutaneous tissues. Many different types of bacteria can cause the infection, and often more than one organism (polymicrobial infection) is to blame. Group A β-haemolytic streptococci however are commonly linked with the disease. The infection can initially be difficult to detect but prompt treatment is essential as mortality rates are high despite aggressive treatment.

A history of trauma or surgery at the affected site is common, however this is not always so (as in our case). Anyone with an infection is theoretically at risk, but in particular the immunocompromised (including diabetics, alcoholics and cancer patients).

Aggressive surgical debridement (often requiring repeated surgical debridement) and intravenous antibiotic therapy, followed by best supportive care, are the mainstay of treatment.

Case 97

A 33-year-old lady presented to accident and emergency complaining of abdominal distension and colicky abdominal pain on and off over the last few days. She had not opened her bowels for four days. She had a long standing history of menorrhagia. Nursing observations were normal, and routine bloods (full blood count, urea and electrolytes) showed a mild microcytic anaemia but were otherwise normal. On examination the abdomen did appear distended, and was fairly firm on palpation, especially in the lower abdomen and pelvis. An abdominal X-ray was requested to rule out obstruction, but the accident and emergency doctor was also concerned about a possible pelvic mass.

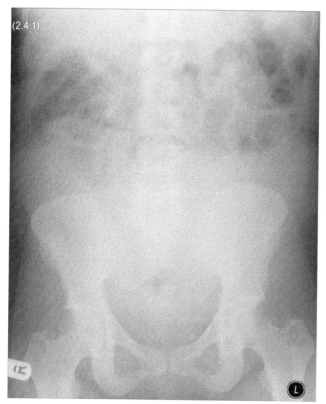

Figure 97.1

Image findings: the abdominal radiograph shows the normal calibre bowel loops have been displaced superiorly into the upper abdomen and there is a paucity of bowel gas in the pelvis and lower abdomen. This suggests that there is a large mass in the pelvis pushing everything out of its way – the superior border of this can just about be made out. There is no evidence of bowel obstruction. Further imaging was requested for further evaluation of the mass lesion.

Given the history of menorrhagia – an MRI was requested.

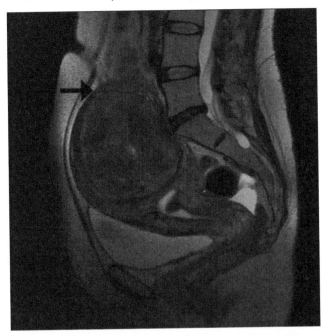

Figure 97.2 MRI showing the superior border of the mass arising from the pelvis (arrow).

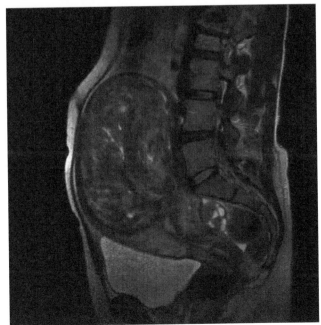

Figure 97.3 T2 weighted sagittal MRI image demonstrates a large well defined round lesion arising from the wall of the uterus which has appearance of a uterine fibroid.

Diagnosis: uterine fibroids.

Uterine fibroids are benign tumours of the uterus characterised by excess growth of smooth muscle cells. They are commoner in Afro-Caribbean women compared to Caucasians by up to five times. Since the tumours are made up of uterine smooth muscle cells they contain oestrogen receptors. This means that the fibroids increase in size during pregnancy and shrink after menopause. For the majority (70%) of cases these are asymptomatic. However, they can present with symptoms of pain, dysmenorrhea, menorrhagia and pressure effects on other pelvic structures, e.g. bladder (urinary frequency) and bowel (constipation).

Fibroids are usually classed according to their position:

- intramural (95%) – confined to the uterine wall. These are most commonly asymptomatic
- subserosal/exophytic (1–2%) – projecting out of the uterine wall
- submucosal (3–4%) – projecting into the endometrial canal.

Major complications include:

- infertility due to narrowing of the fallopian tubes
- complication in pregnancy, e.g. spontaneous abortions, ectopic pregnancies, placental abruption, intrauterine growth restriction
- malignant transformation (very rare – 0.2%).

There are several methods of treatment which include hysterectomy and uterine artery embolisation.

Case 98

A 70-year-old woman presents to the emergency department following a twisting injury to her left foot and ankle. Clinical examination reveals tenderness over the fifth metatarsal. A radiograph of the left foot is requested.

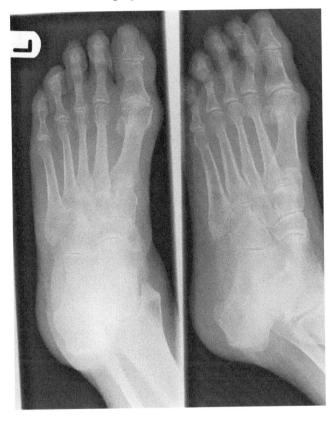

Figure 98.1

Image findings: there is a transverse avulsion fracture at the base of the fifth metatarsal with minimal displacement of the fracture fragments.

Diagnosis: an avulsion fracture at the base of the fifth metatarsal.

Fractures at the base of the fifth metatarsal are one of the most common injuries encountered in the emergency department. The peroneus brevis tendon inserts at the tuberosity of the base of the fifth metatarsal and an avulsion fracture occurs as a result of forced inversion of the foot in plantar flexion (e.g. stepping off a curb). Clinical examination usually demonstrates swelling and focal tenderness at the base of the fifth metatarsal. As for all fractures, a plain radiograph should be the first line investigation.

Care should be taken when diagnosing an avulsion fracture in children as a secondary ossification centre (apophysis) may be seen at the base of the fifth metatarsal which may simulate a fracture. As a rule of thumb, avulsion fractures tend to have a transverse/horizontal fracture line and may extend into the joint. In contrast the apophysis of a secondary ossification centre will be longitudinal and parallel to the shaft of the metatarsal, *see* Figure 98.2, smoothly corticated and never extend into the joint.

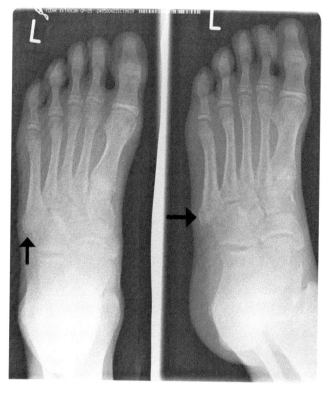

Figure 98.2 AP and oblique views of the foot demonstrates the appearance of a normal apophysis and should not be mistaken for a fracture (arrow).

The term Jones fracture is used to describe a transverse fracture of the proximal shaft of the fifth metatarsal. An avulsion fracture at the base of the fifth metatarsal is frequently referred to as a pseudo-Jones fracture.

Case 99

A 13-year-old boy is seen in the emergency department following a fall from a ladder during gymnastics. Clinical examination reveals swelling and tenderness overlying the proximal tibia. A radiograph of the knee is requested.

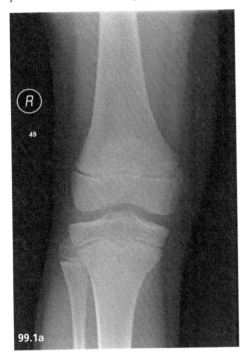

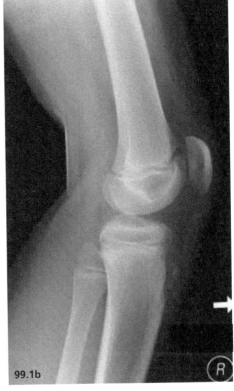

Figures 99.1a, b

Image findings: this is an AP and lateral view of the right knee. There is fragmentation of the tibial tuberosity. There is also soft tissue swelling overlying the tibial tuberosity with thickening of the distal patellar tendon.

Diagnosis: Osgood-Schlatter disease.

Osgood-Schlatter disease is a common cause of knee pain in young active patients and occurs during a period of rapid growth when the tibial tubercle is maturing. It is more common in males and usually presents between 10–15 years of age. The classical clinical presentation is of anterior knee ache which worsens with activity. There is usually tenderness and swelling around the patella tendon and tibial tuberosity.

The multiple ossification centres anterior to the tibial tuberosity seen in Osgood-Schlatter disease occurs as a result of repeated microtrauma in the deep fibres of the patella tendon at the site of its insertion with the tibial tuberosity. An avulsion of the patellar tendon may also be present. However the appearance of multiple ossification centres at the tibial tubercle, anterior to the tibial metaphysis can also be a normal variant, especially if there is no associated tenderness or swelling.

Osgood-Schlatter disease is managed with rest from strenuous activities, analgesia and non-steroidal anti-inflammatory drugs. Surgery is reserved for patients that do not improve with conservative management. The surgical options include debulking or excision of the tibial tuberosity.

Case 100

A 30-year-old man was stabbed in the right side of the chest. He presented to the emergency department with chest and upper abdominal pain. An erect chest radiograph was performed.

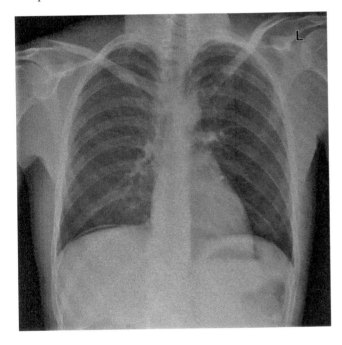

Figure 100.1

Image findings: the erect chest X-ray shows free air beneath the right hemidiaphragm, also termed pneumoperitoneum, which refers to the presence of air within the peritoneal cavity.

Diagnosis: pneumoperitoneum.

In this patient, the free air was due to perforated bowel from the knife injury. The most common cause of pneumoperitoneum is perforation of an abdominal viscus, most commonly, a perforated ulcer, although a pneumoperitoneum may occur as a result of perforation of any part of the bowel – for example, a perforated malignant colonic tumor, appendix rupture, bowel inflammation, e.g. inflammatory bowel disease, or a diverticulum. Pneumoperitoneum can also be due to infection of the peritoneal cavity with a gas forming organism; iatrogenic causes such as recent surgery or trauma, bowel obstruction (gas permeates through the bowel wall) and extension from the chest, e.g. pnemomediastinum.

It should be remembered that following surgery (both open and laparoscopic), a small amount of free intra-peritoneal air will be a normal finding, but this should be absorbed within 3–5 days.

Free intraperitoneal gas on a supine abdominal radiograph gives signs of:

- **Rigler's sign** – air is seen outlining the wall of the bowel since there is both gas inside and outside the bowel, *see* Figures 100.2 and 100.3
- **triangle sign** – air in an abdominal viscus will not form straight edges but free intraperitoneal air does
- **football sign** – large lucency in the centre of the abdomen since air is lighter than fat and rises to the anterior aspect.

Pneumoperitoneum is an emergency and *immediate* referral to the surgical team is required. CT abdomen can be useful to look for the cause of free gas and also to look for other associated injuries, e.g. in this case to exclude a liver laceration.

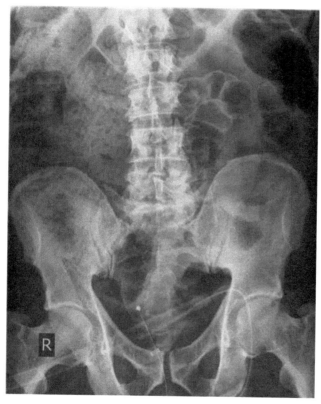

Figure 100.2

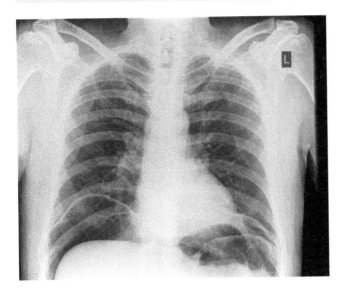

Figure 100.3

Figures 100.2 and 100.3 are abdominal and chest radiographs of a patient who was one-day post surgery (a post surgical drain is still seen in situ at the bottom of the film). The radiographs demonstrate Rigler's sign – with pneumoperitoneum in this case being as a consequence of the recent surgery and the drain still being in situ.

Index

T - #1040 - 101024 - C0 - 246/171/16 - PB - 9781846194528 - Gloss Lamination